Chronic Pain: the Occupational

For Churchill Livingstone:

Editorial director: Mary Law
Project development editor: Mairi McCubbin
Project manager: Valerie Burgess
Project controller: Pat Miller
Copy editor: Stephanie Pickering
Indexer: Nina Boyd
Design direction: Judith Wright
Sales promotion executive: Maria O'Connor

Chronic Pain: the Occupational Therapist's Perspective

Jennifer Strong PhD
Senior Lecturer, Department of Occupational Therapy,
The University of Queensland, Australia

Foreword by

Robert G. Large MB ChB PhD FRANZCP
Chairperson of the Auckland Regional Pain Service,
New Zealand

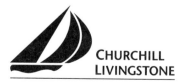

NEW YORK EDINBURGH LONDON MADRID MELBOURNE SAN FRANCISCO TOKYO 1996

CHURCHILL LIVINGSTONE
Medical Division of Pearson Professional Limited

Distributed in the United States of America by Churchill Livingstone, 650 Avenue of the Americas, New York, N.Y. 10011, and by associated companies, branches and representatives throughout the world.

© Pearson Professional Limited 1996

All rights reserved. No part of this publication may be reproduced, stored in a retrieval system, or transmitted in any form or by any means, electronic, mechanical, photocopying, recording or otherwise, without either the prior permission of the publishers (Churchill Livingstone, Robert Stevenson House, 1-3 Baxter's Place, Leith Walk, Edinburgh, EH1 3AF), or a licence permitting restricted copying in the United Kingdom issued by the Copyright Licensing Agency Ltd, 90 Tottenham Court Road, London, W1P 9HE.

First published 1996

ISBN   0 443 05251 4

British Library Cataloguing in Publication Data
A catalogue record for this book is available from the British Library.

Library of Congress Cataloging in Publication Data
A catalog record for this book is available from the Library of Congress.

Note
Medical knowledge is constantly changing. As new information becomes available, changes in treatment, procedures, equipment and the use of drugs become necessary. The editors/authors/contributors and the publishers have, as far as it is possible, taken care to ensure that the information given in this text is accurate and up to date. However, readers are strongly advised to confirm that the information, especially with regard to drug usage, complies with latest legislation and standards of practice.

The publisher's policy is to use **paper manufactured from sustainable forests**

Produced through Longman Malaysia, PP

Contents

Foreword   vii
Preface   ix

SECTION 1 Background   1
1. Explaining pain   3
2. Epidemiology of chronic pain   13
3. Models for intervention   29

SECTION 2 Occupational therapy concerns   41
4. Occupational therapy involvement in pain management   43
5. Assessment issues   71
6. Scope of occupational therapy treatment   93
7. Treatment issues–techniques for pain management   117
8. Special treatment topics   139

SECTION 3 Synthesis   153
9. Synthesis   155

Index   165

Foreword

Pain is full of paradoxes! As an ubiquitous human experience, we all assume that we know what it is. However, it is hard to define and measure.

Acute pain is experienced at some time by most people, so we extrapolate from those experiences in our attempts to understand chronic pain; yet chronic pain is vastly different from acute pain. So much so that it requires different explanatory models and treatment approaches.

Chronic non-cancer pain has sometimes been called 'benign', despite being a potent cause of human misery and disability. The struggle to deal with chronic pain has stimulated the development of multidisciplinary approaches to care. However, the disciplines have been slow to develop a truly 'interdisciplinary' approach, as espoused in this book.

Medical specialties, psychology and physiotherapy have tended to dominate the literature on pain management, and there is an increasing recognition by these disciplines of the impact of pain on activity and function. It is very likely that this recognition has sprung from the work of the many occupational therapists who have contributed to multidisciplinary pain clinics without, necessarily, writing of their experience in pain journals.

This book begins to redress the balance. Jenny Strong is a clinical and academic occupational therapist who has made substantial contributions to the literature on chronic pain. She writes with the authority of one who knows the clinical realities of pain as well as understanding the requirements of clinical research.

Occupational therapists will find this book a friendly guide to the fascinating and demanding world of pain management; just as readers from other disciplines (and hopefully, clinical directors of pain clinics!) will discover the debt they owe to occupational therapy. All readers will be excited by the therapeutic possibilities which are encouraged by the vision of a discipline which focuses so clearly on the things which matter in daily living.

Auckland, 1996   R. G. L.

Preface

As recently as 1990, Nanci I Moore commented that: 'Few descriptions of pain teams include the role of the occupational therapist'. Such lack of visibility of occupational therapy could be due to occupational therapists playing a less than active role in both the treatment and management of individuals with chronic pain, and the research function of the pain team, and as such, have not rated a mention as a core team member. Certainly, it has only been in the last decade that occupational therapists have begun to document their involvement in this practice area. My own writings on occupational therapy and pain have shown my own developmental progression; moving from the delineation of occupational therapy services to documentation about practice extent, to education of other health professionals about the occupational therapy role, to treatment efficacy studies, and the refinement of measurement systems.

Despite the increase in occupational therapy literature on pain management, there remains a general lack of appreciation of how occupational therapists may assist the person with pain. Such a lack of general acknowledgement of the occupational therapy contribution in pain management has been one of the stimuli for writing this book. Another indirect purpose of the book is to inform other members of pain teams about the occupational therapy role in pain management.

The book has been written to provide a guide for both practising occupational therapists and occupational therapy students who may be contemplating working with people with pain in a variety of practice settings, such as pain clinics, general hospitals, paediatric hospitals, nursing homes or hospice services. There is, from my observation and experience, much work for occupational therapists in the area of pain management. Rather than teaching occupational therapists who are starting at the beginning and inventing their own wheel, this book has been designed to circumvent such duplication of effort, so that more energy can be directed towards increasing the momentum, direction and accuracy of our wheel. The book attempts to synthesize knowledge from the fields of current pain management practices and occupational therapy practice. The book is by no means a definitive textbook on pain, and throughout the text the reader is referred to other seminal works in the pain area.

Section 1 of the book begins by defining terms so that our goals may be clearer when reading the book. Who are we talking about when we say 'a patient with chronic pain?' How does acute pain differ from chronic pain? How is pain felt? In Chapter 1, questions such as these are considered. In the second chapter, an attempt is made to delineate the extent of the problem of chronic pain in the community. An examination is made of the available epidemiological studies which have attempted to map chronic pain in the community. Having drawn a picture of both the problems faced by the person with chronic pain, and the extent of the problem in our community, Chapter 3 then provides an overview of models for managing and treating people with chronic pain.

Section 2 of the book begins with Chapter 4, where an examination is made of occupational therapy models of practice for pain management. Then the practice model which I have found to be useful in my own work is outlined and illustrated. The unique and valuable contribution which the occupational therapist can make to the person with pain is thus unveiled in this chapter. Occupational therapists must be as sure as they can that their interventions are based upon good art and science. Assessments must be reliable and valid, and treatments efficacious. Chapter 5 examines pain assessment practices in some detail, with the emphasis upon multidimensional assessment. Chapters 6 and 7 are concerned with treatment. Chapter 6 examines treatment from the work, self-care and leisure perspectives, while Chapter 7 considers a variety of treatment techniques. Case examples are used to illustrate salient points. Chapter 8 then considers the special topics of pain in children, the elderly and those with cancer.

Upon reaching the final chapter (Chapter 9), it is to be hoped that the reader will be excited about what the occupational therapist is able to contribute to the area of pain management. In Chapter 9, a synthesis is made of the material presented in the book.

I would like to acknowledge the assistance I have received from a number of sources while preparing this book: The University of Queensland for providing me with Special Studies Leave, The University of Auckland for providing me with shelter and a stimulating environment, and the New Zealand Government for awarding me an ANZAC Fellowship in 1993. My husband, Paul Nutt, deserves my special thanks, for his encouragement, support and infinite patience. Judy Waters is to be thanked for her excellent advice to the novice author. Finally, I would like to thank the many people with pain, with whom I have worked, for teaching me, firsthand, the value of occupation.

1996   J. S.

SECTION 1

Background

Section 1 begins with definitions of terms. This is followed by delineation of the extent of the pain problem and then by presentation of models for the management of pain.

SECTION CONTENTS

1. Explaining pain 3

2. Epidemiology of chronic pain 13

3. Models for intervention 29

1

Explaining pain

Defining pain 4
Acute pain and chronic pain 5
  Characteristics of the chronic pain
    syndrome 6
  Cancer and non-cancer pain 7
Clinical pain states 7
  Nociceptive pain 7
  Neuropathic pain 7
  Psychogenic pain 7

Pain perception 8
  Variables influencing pain
    perception 8
  How is pain perceived? 8
  The gate control theory of pain 9
  The modified gate control theory of
    pain 10
Chapter summary 10
References 10

The thesis of this book is that pain, and in particular chronic pain, is a problem large enough to concern occupational therapists, due to its considerable impact on the occupational performance of many individuals. Increasingly, many occupational therapists are realizing that pain is a major problem for their patients, and that expertise is needed to manage it; yet there is a dearth of books on the subject of occupational therapy and chronic pain. Only one collection of papers, *Occupational therapy and the patient with pain* (Cromwell 1984) has appeared; no other books are available specifically for the occupational therapist.

Many people with pain can benefit from the assistance of occupational therapists, but we must be careful not to jump into the water before we examine the pond – we need to be well versed in what causes intractable pain, its extent in our communities, how it affects the individual, how it can be quantified and the current management models. Then, we need to be clear, articulate and skilled in order to provide the most appropriate and efficacious occupational therapy service for people in pain.

This chapter explains why it is necessary to have a book on occupational therapy and pain, and why pain needs consideration as an entity in its own right. After all, there are books aplenty on topics such as arthritis (which has the frequent concomitant of pain) and on pain in general. Why occupational therapy and pain?

We need to draw a picture of the person with a chronic pain problem in order to see how the occupational therapist fits into it. Occupational therapists looking at this picture may think, 'This person's life has been greatly affected by his pain experience. With my skills, I could help the individual to improve his quality of life by ... '. There are a great many pain services which do valuable work in assisting patients with chronic pain problems. Some of these services do not have occupational therapy involvement. I have observed such services and acknowledged the contribution they make, but at the same time, I have often wondered if the patients concerned could have benefited even more by being seen also by an occupational therapist.

We will begin by defining the phenomenon of pain. Then, we will look at the differences between acute pain and chronic pain, and examine the characteristics of what is known as the chronic pain syndrome. An alternative clinical classification of pain conditions based on underlying pain pathophysiology will then be reviewed. Consideration will be given to variables which influence an individual's pain perception. A brief examination will be made of pain perception, and consideration given to the gate control theory of pain.

DEFINING PAIN

There is no single universally accepted definition of pain (Elton et al 1983, Melzack & Wall 1982). If we enlist the help of a dictionary, we find that the word 'pain' is derived from the Latin word *poena*, which means punishment or penalty. The *Oxford Reference Dictionary* (1986, cited in Bendelow 1993) defines pain as:

1. an unpleasant feeling caused by injury or disease of the body
2. mental suffering
3. [old use] punishment, e.g. on pain of death.

The McGraw Hill *Dictionary of Scientific and Technical Terms* defines pain as 'patterns of somesthetic sensation, generally unpleasant, or causing suffering or distress'.

In gaining a more complete understanding of the word 'pain', we find that its antonym is 'pleasure'. So, to have pain is clearly a bad thing, to be avoided if at all possible.

Rey (1993) has translated a pertinent Latin text:

Every living being from its very moment of birth seeks pleasure, enjoying it as the ultimate good while rejecting pain as the ultimate adversity and, insofar as is possible, doing his best to avoid it; he behaves in this fashion to the extent that he has not yet been conditioned and insofar as his basic nature has been left intact to judge naturally and with integrity.

Perhaps the most widely accepted definition of pain is that provided by the International Association for the Study of Pain (IASP), which describes pain as: 'An unpleasant sensory and emotional experience associated with actual or potential tissue damage, or described in terms of such damage' (IASP 1979, Merskey 1986). This definition acknowledges that pain can and does exist in the absence of direct tissue insult or nociception.

Clearly, there is a biological imperative to remove oneself from the stimulus of pain, or to eliminate the pain. Such an action can be as simple as removing one's hand from the lighted hotplate. Another imperative is to alleviate the pain at the site of injury. This can be achieved by such actions as plunging the hand into cool water or by vigorously shaking the hand. In acute pain situations, much can often be done to alleviate the pain and prevent suffering. But what of the situation when the pain is chronic? Human beings still have the desire to eliminate or reduce the pain.

Let us think for a moment of head pain, or as it is more commonly known, headache. Now, if I have a headache for a few hours, I may be inconvenienced enough to take some sort of headache preparation (medication). If this headache were to linger for the whole day, I might begin to feel out of sorts and a bit grumpy. If I did not sleep much that night because of the headache, and arose in the morning with the headache still there, it is highly probable that I would not be able to concentrate properly on my normal activities of daily living. It is also likely that I would begin to see the headache as a sinister symptom of some serious disease. I would most likely visit the doctor, both to obtain relief from the headache and to check what was causing it. If the doctor were to tell me that she could not find any cause for the headache, and that I just had to put up with it, then it is likely that I would take myself off to another doctor who could help me. I would be feeling some despair by this time. If my headache were to continue, day in and day out, for days, weeks, months or years, I am sure that all aspects of my life would be severely affected. My work would suffer, my interpersonal relationships would deteriorate, my leisure time would be ruined and the performance of my personal and instrumental activities of daily living would become perfunctory and patchy.

In this situation, and that of other chronic pain conditions, I am reminded of the words of Emily Dickinson, who said 'Pain has an element of blank it cannot recollect when it began — or if there were a time when it was not — It has no Future but itself — Its Infinite realms contain Its Past — enlightened to perceive New Periods — of Pain'.

Dickinson's words capture the overwhelming, all-encompassing nature of the chronic pain phenomenon. Or, as Melzack (1990) puts it, 'Prolonged pain destroys the quality of life'.

Let us now look at the distinction between acute pain and chronic pain.

ACUTE PAIN AND CHRONIC PAIN

In recent years, chronic pain has emerged as a phenomenon distinct from acute pain (Merskey 1986). Acute pain serves as an important mechanism to warn the body of injury or disease (Cailliet 1979), and its characteristics include tissue damage, pain and anxiety (Sternbach 1974). Chronic pain, however, differs from acute pain in a number of ways; it persists, constantly or intermittently, past the normal time of healing (Sternbach 1974), and it serves no useful biological purpose to the individual (Little 1981).

The time at which persisting pain is termed 'chronic' may vary from 1 month to 6 months (Merskey 1986). (The IASP considers the demarcation point between acute and chronic pain to be 3 months (Merskey 1986).) Four frequently occurring components of chronic pain are (Cailliet 1979):

- nociception (tissue irritation)
- pain transmission in the central nervous system
- suffering (the individual's affective response to the pain)
- pain behaviour.

Chronic pain will affect the person as a whole and is not confined to the painful body part (Rey 1993).

Characteristics of the chronic pain syndrome

Chronic pain which persists past the time of normal healing can be considered as a pain syndrome (Little 1981, Melzack & Wall 1982). Patients with chronic pain may exhibit a number of the characteristics listed in Box 1.1.

Clearly then, when we think about an individual with chronic pain, we are most probably thinking about a person who has major difficulties in multiple facets of his life. Many such difficulties (occupational role disruption, psychosocial withdrawal, feelings of helplessness, loss of self-esteem and physical incapacity, for example) are in areas where occupational therapists have developed considerable skills in providing assistance to the individual.

Box 1.1 Chronic pain characteristics

1. A poor response to conventional analgesia (Sternbach 1974).
2. Multiple surgical and/or pharmacological treatments (Pinsky et al 1979).
3. An increase in help-seeking behaviours (Sternbach 1974).
4. Mood and affect changes (Pinsky et al 1979).
5. An increase in feelings of helplessness, hopelessness and meaninglessness (Sternbach 1974).
6. Escalating psychosocial withdrawal (Pinsky et al 1979).
7. Disruptions in occupational role performance (Roy 1984, Strong 1986).
8. A decrease in self-esteem (Pinsky et al 1979).
9. Escalating physical incapacity due to disuse (Pinsky et al 1979).
10. Conflicts with health care providers (Pinsky et al 1979).

Cancer and non-cancer pain

An important distinction needs to be made here between chronic pain of cancer and non-cancer origin (Sternbach 1974). The management of these two types of chronic pain is quite different. The main goal of treatment for the patient with cancer pain is to relieve the pain, while the main goal of treatment for the patient with non-cancer pain is to assist the individual to live with the pain as a functional human being. Apart from an overview of cancer pain management (Ch. 3) and the special topics section on cancer pain in Chapter 8, the remainder of this book will refer primarily to non-cancer pain, unless otherwise indicated in the text.

CLINICAL PAIN STATES

In addition to the acute/chronic classification, another frequently used clinical classification system recognizes three types of pain based upon the underlying pathophysiology of the pain. These pains are nociceptive pain, neuropathic pain and psychogenic pain (Andersson & Yokola 1987, Portenoy 1989).

Nociceptive pain

Nociceptive pain may be either somatic or visceral in origin, and is considered to be pain which relates to the stimulation of nociceptive pathways (Portenoy 1989). Nociceptive pain includes arthritic pain and most cancer pain (Portenoy 1989).

Neuropathic pain

Neuropathic pain arises from injuries to neural structures (Portenoy 1989). It includes deafferentation pain, sympathetically maintained pain and peripheral pain (Portenoy 1989). Deafferentation pain is due to central neurone activity (for example, brachial plexus avulsion lesion pain); sympathetically maintained pain is due to activity in the sympathetic nervous system efferents (for example, reflex sympathetic dystrophy); while peripheral pain is due to mechanisms such as the abnormal sprouting of injured nerves (to cause a neuroma) (Portenoy 1989).

Psychogenic pain

Psychogenic or idiopathic pain is the term used for pain states where no organic lesion can be found, or where the pain complaint is considered to be out of proportion to the organic pathology (Portenoy 1989). Of all the pain classifications, it is psychogenic pain which causes the most distress and anger in the patient. Many workers have suggested that it should not be used as a classification. The typical story related by patients is as follows: 'I went to this specialist and she examined me, told me there was nothing wrong with me and that the pain was all in my head. I had psychogenic pain'. All types of pain are ultimately perceived in one's head; and, as this book will demonstrate, many pains have associated psychological concomitants, be they precedents or antecedents of the pain.

PAIN PERCEPTION

Before we look at pain perception in more detail, we should be aware of the variables which influence the individual's response to painful stimuli.

Variables influencing pain perception

People vary in their responses to painful stimuli of seemingly equal magnitude. A good contemporary example of this would be the ability of sportsmen and sportswomen to continue with the game despite tissue damage which would cause considerable pain to a non-player. One has only to think of footballers on the football field or competitors in an ironman series to illustrate this point. Only after the game is over do the footballers experience the pain associated with tissue damage. A more historical example would be soldiers on the battlefield who, despite severe injuries, continued to fight to save their lives – only after the danger had passed did they perceive the pain (Beecher 1957).

How is pain perceived?

It is important for occupational therapists to have an understanding of how a person perceives pain. It is also important to keep abreast of new findings in the area. Our understanding of pain continues to grow, thanks to the contributions of both the basic and the clinical sciences. I can remember the feelings of excitement I experienced at my first World Congress on Pain. So much was happening, but how could I ever understand it all and keep abreast of the accumulating knowledge? It is certainly not necessary for the occupational therapist to know all there is to know in the areas of pain neuroanatomy, pain neurophysiology and pain biochemistry. However, we do need a certain level of knowledge and understanding. I still smart at the memory of a meeting I attended between occupational therapists and another health professional group working in pain, during which an occupational therapist (who worked in a pain clinic) betrayed a total lack of awareness of the gate control theory of pain – a theory which has been 'the most influential and important current theory of pain perception' (Weisenberg 1977).

So, let us look at some of the aspects of pain perception. We will review the gate control theory of pain proposed by Melzack and Wall (1965). We will briefly at what happens at the periphery, in the spinal cord and in the central nervous system. For a more complete coverage of the underlying anatomical and physiological basis of pain, the interested reader is referred in the first instance to chapters in Wall and Melzack's *Textbook of Pain* (1989, 1994).

The gate control theory of pain

The gate control theory of pain, developed by Melzack and Wall (1965) proposed that there exists in the dorsal horn of the spinal cord, a gate-like mechanism which can be opened or shut to peripheral nerve impulses trying to get to the brain. The dorsal horn substantia gelatinosa cells were considered to be the neural structure which controlled this gate (Melzack & Wall 1982). Impulses allowed through the gate by the substantia gelatinosa neurones were relayed to the transmission cells (T cells) in the dorsal horn for central projection.

At the periphery can be found two sorts of small diameter nerve fibres – A-delta fibres and C fibres (Weisenberg 1977). The A-delta fibres or Type II AMH nociceptors, sensitive to noxious mechanical impulses, pick up short latency pricking-type pain. The unmyelinated C fibres, sensitive to mechanical, thermal and chemical noxious stimuli, pick up long latency burning pain (Cervero 1986).

The C fibres are known as polymodal nociceptors (Campbell et al 1989). Also in the periphery are large diameter A-beta fibres which are cutaneous mechanoreceptors (Bowsher 1988a, Cervero 1986), known as Type I AMH nociceptors (Campbell et al 1989).

The gate control theory hypothesizes that the small diameter fibres act to inhibit the substantia gelatinosa neurones, which then open the gate and thereby facilitate T-cell activity (and pain), while the large diameter fibres facilitate the substantia gelatinosa neurones to close the gate and prevent T-cell transmission of nociception (that is, shutting the gate).

Within the central nervous system are a number of structures relevant to pain perception. Impulses from the T cells of the spinal cord ascend along the contralateral anterolateral quadrant. One of the major tracts of the anterolateral system is the spinothalamic tract (Cervero 1986), which is the primary nociceptive pathway in the spinal cord (Willis 1989). Impulses are projected to the brain stem reticular activating formation, the tectum, the ventral posterior lateral nuclei and the central lateral nuclei of the intralaminar complex of the thalamus, the periaqueductal grey matter of the upper brain stem, and the somatosensory cortex (Bowsher 1988b, Cervero 1986, Willis 1989). Many parts of the cerebral cortex have been shown to have increased metabolism following painful stimulation (Cervero 1986).

The modified gate control theory of pain

In the face of advancing knowledge, Melzack and Wall (1982) made a number of modifications to the gate control theory of pain: in particular, they acknowledged the importance of an inhibitory brainstem system which projects down into the dorsal horn of the spinal cord, as well as the possible excitatory and inhibitory functions of the substantia gelatinosa cells.

This theory has helped to make enormous inroads into both our understanding and our management of pain. On a clinical level, the theory has been valuable in terms of management practices such as non-painful stimulation, cognitive techniques, activity engagement and behavioural techniques, that is, methods which focus upon activating pain inhibiting mechanisms. The theory's acknowledgement of the multidimensional nature of the pain experience, incorporating as it does the sensory, cognitive and affective dimensions of pain, has also been of enormous value (Turk et al 1983). At the basic science level, the theory provided the structure for testable hypotheses about the anatomy and physiology of pain (Hoffert 1989). From the flurry of research in the area, much of 'the original gate control theory has been disproved' (Hoffert 1989): aspects in question include the role of the substantia gelatinosa in gating, and the mechanisms for the inhibition of the afferent impulses (Anonymous 1978, Nathan 1976). Yet, in lieu of another clearly enunciated theory which takes on board the research advances, it remains a useful heuristic guide. I find it particularly useful in explaining the pain experience to patients, linking as it does the sensory, affective and cognitive components of pain.

CHAPTER SUMMARY

In this chapter, we have explored what pain is: how it is defined, the types of pain which exist, the characteristics of the chronic pain syndrome, and how pain is perceived. Such a grounding is essential for occupational therapists wishing to help individuals with pain problems. We will now turn to the next important question: how big is the pain problem? In the next chapter, we will consider the epidemiological data which map out the size of the pain problem.

REFERENCES

Andersson S, Yokola T 1987 Anatomical, pathophysiological and biochemical aspects of pain. In: Andersson S, Bond M, Mehta M, Swerdlow M (eds) Chronic non-cancer pain assessment and practical management. MTP Press, Lancaster

Anonymous 1978 The gate control theory of pain. British Medical Journal 2: 586–587

Beecher H K 1957 The measurement of pain. Pharmacological Reviews 9: 59–209
Bendelow G 1993 Pain perceptions, emotions and gender. Sociology of Health and Illness 15: 273–296
Bowsher D 1988a Nociceptors and peripheral nerve fibres. In: Wells P E, Frampton V, Bowsher D (eds) Pain management and control in physiotherapy. Heinemann, London
Bowsher D 1988b Central pain mechanisms. In: Wells P E, Frampton V, Bowsher D (eds) Pain management and control in physiotherapy. Heinemann, London
Cailliet R 1979 Chronic pain: is it necessary? Archives of Physical Medicine and Rehabilitation 60: 4–7
Campbell J N, Raja S N, Cohen R H, Manning D C, Khan A A, Meyer R A 1989 Peripheral neural mechanisms of nociception. In: Wall P D, Melzack R (eds) Textbook of pain, 2nd edn. Churchill Livingstone, Edinburgh
Cervero F 1986 Neurophysiological aspects of pain and pain therapy. In: Swerdlow M (ed) The therapy of pain, 2nd edn. MTP Press, Lancaster
Cromwell F S (ed) 1984 Occupational therapy and the patient with pain. Haworth Press, Binghamton, NY and Occupational Therapy in Health Care 1: 3
Dictionary of scientific and technical terms. McGraw Hill
Elton D, Stanley G, Burrows G 1983 Psychological control of pain. Grune & Stratton, Sydney
Hoffert M J 1989 The neurophysiology of pain. Neurologic Clinics 7: 183–203
International Association for the Study of Pain 1979 Pain terms: a list with definitions and notes on usage. Pain 6: 249–252
Little T F 1981 Chronic pain. Modern concepts in management. Australian Family Physician 10: 265–270
Melzack R 1990 The tragedy of needless pain. Scientific American 262: 19–25
Melzack R, Wall P D 1965 Pain mechanisms: a new theory. Science 150: 971–976
Melzack R, Wall P D 1982 The challenge of pain. Penguin Books, Harmondsworth
Merskey H (ed) 1986 Classification of chronic pain. Descriptions of chronic pain syndromes and definitions of pain terms. Pain 24(3): S1–S211
Nathan P W 1976 The gate-control theory of pain: a critical review. Brain 99: 123–158
Oxford reference dictionary 1986 Oxford
Pinsky J J, Griffin S E, Agnew D C, Kamdar M D, Crue B L, Pinsky L H 1979 Aspects of long-term evaluation of pain unit treatment programs for patients with chronic intractable benign pain syndrome: treatment outcome. Bulletin Los Angeles Neurological Society 44: 53–69
Portenoy R K 1989 Mechanisms of clinical pain: observations and speculations. Neurologic Clinics 7: 205–230
Rey R 1993 History of pain. Editions la Découverte, Paris
Roy R 1984 Pain clinics: reassessment of objectives and outcomes. Archives of Physical Medicine and Rehabilitation 65: 448–451
Sternbach R A 1974 Pain patients traits and treatment. Academic Press, New York
Strong J 1986 Occupational therapy and chronic pain. Proceedings of the 8th Annual Scientific Meeting, Australian Pain Society, Melbourne
Turk D C, Meichenbaum D, Genest M 1983 Pain and behavioral medicine. A cognitive–behavioral perspective. Guilford Press, New York
Wall P D 1978 The gate control theory of pain mechanisms: A re-examination and re-statement. Brain 101: 1–18
Wall P D 1989 The dorsal horn. In: Wall P D, Melzack R (eds) Textbook of pain, 2nd edn. Churchill Livingstone, Edinburgh
Wall P D, Melzack R (eds) 1989 Textbook of pain, 2nd edn. Churchill Livingstone, Edinburgh
Wall P D, Melzack R (eds) 1994 Textbook of pain, 3rd edn. Churchill Livingstone, Edinburgh
Weisenberg M 1977 Pain and pain control. Psychological Bulletin 84: 1008–1044
Willis W D 1989 The origin and destination of pathways involved in pain transmission. In: Wall P D, Melzack R (eds) Textbook of pain, 2nd edn. Churchill Livingstone, Edinburgh

2

Epidemiology of chronic pain

Definition of terms 14	**Natural history of pain** 21
Definitions in pain surveys 14	**Aetiological factors in developing**
Aspects of pain epidemiology 14	**chronic pain** 22
Extent of the pain problem 15	Back pain – risk factors 22
Australia 16	**Summary of epidemiological**
Canada 16	**findings** 23
Great Britain 17	**Implications for occupational**
New Zealand 17	**therapists** 24
Scandinavia 18	**Chapter summary** 25
United States of America 19	**References** 25
General reviews 21	

Epidemiological research seeks to study chronic pain in populations as a dynamic process characterised by the integrated action of agent, host, and environmental factors (Von Korff 1992).

Chronic pain is a debilitating and expensive condition, expensive both in terms of human suffering to individuals and their families and in terms of the financial cost to individuals, families and communities. How exactly do we go about getting an indication of the size of this problem? In this chapter, we will examine the available literature in an attempt to define the extent of the problem of chronic pain in our communities. It will be particularly helpful to look at the epidemiological literature. Epidemiology has been defined as 'the study of the factors determining the frequency and distribution of disease [in this case, chronic pain] in human populations' (Lowe & Kostrzewski 1973). Like the aims of epidemiology identified by Lowe and Kostrzewski (1973), this chapter will attempt to go some way towards describing the distribution and size of the chronic pain problem, identifying aetiological factors in the development of chronic pain problems in human individuals, and providing data necessary for the planning of services (in this case, occupational therapy services for people with chronic pain).

It should be noted at the outset that much remains to be done to gain a complete picture of the magnitude and extent of chronic pain in our community. As Crombie and his colleagues (1994) noted: 'the published studies tell us only a little about the nature of the public health problem [of chronic pain]'. However, we will address the question to the best of our ability. We begin by looking at a definition of terms, and then consider the extent of the pain problem, the natural history of pain, and aetiological factors in the development of chronic pain problems. Finally, the relevance of such information to occupational therapists will be discussed.

DEFINITION OF TERMS

'The epidemiological literature on chronic pain ... suffers from a lack of consensus about basic definitions and from inconsistencies in measurement which make it difficult to compare studies and to generate precise numbers' (Osterweis et al 1987). Despite the problem of definition, we can say with some certainty that the experience of persistent pain is a common one (Croft et al 1993).

As we discussed in Chapter 1, we must begin by providing some clear definitions of the phenomena with which we are concerned. As mentioned in Chapter 1, the International Association for the Study of Pain has defined pain as: 'An unpleasant sensory and emotional experience associated with actual or potential tissue damage, or described in terms of such damage' (Merskey 1986). Chronic pain is considered to be pain which exists past the 'normal time of healing', and the IASP has defined the time after which acute pain becomes chronic pain as 3 months (IASP, cited in Merskey 1986).

Definitions in pain surveys

With these definitions in mind, let us now also look at how pain surveys have defined the terms. Differences do exist in how pain has been defined (Crombie et al 1994, Osterweis et al 1987). For example, Crook et al (1984) asked respondents 'Are you or any members of your family over 18 years of age *often* troubled with pain? Have you or any family member experienced any noteworthy pain within the past 2 weeks?' Subjects who reported being troubled with pain often and within the past 2 weeks were then classified as having persistent pain. James et al (1991), however, recorded pain prevalence only if subjects had ever experienced pain severe enough to lead to a consultation with a doctor or other health professional, or where it led to the use of medication for pain which was taken more than once, or where the pain interfered with life or activities 'a lot'. Meanwhile, Croft et al (1993) defined pain as 'A report of any pain during the past month which had lasted for longer than 24 hours', and chronic pain as 'Pain, as defined above, which had started more than 3 months ago'.

Aspects of pain epidemiology

Aspects of pain which can be studied epidemiologically include pain prevalence, pain incidence, natural history, relative risk factors, prognosis, and the relationships between prevalence, incidence and duration (Von Korff 1992). The most frequently considered aspects of pain epidemiology have been its incidence and prevalence.

Pain incidence

Pain incidence refers to the rate of onset of pain amongst individuals with no previous history of pain (Von Korff 1992). However, once again, the term has been used differently in different pain surveys. For example, Osterweis et al (1987) have defined incidence as the 'number of new cases of the pain problem occurring in the population during a specified period of time', whereas Spitzer et al (1987) defined incidence as 'the proportion of workers who were compensated with absence from work of at least 1 day, for a spinal disorder at least one time during 1981, regardless of the number of times'. These two examples come from slightly different contexts, but nevertheless also have slightly different meanings.

Pain prevalence

Pain prevalence can refer to point prevalence rates or lifetime prevalence rates (Von Korff 1992). Most pain studies have considered the point prevalence rate, which is defined as the 'total number of cases of condition present in the population at a particular time'.

Natural history of pain

Measures of the natural history of pain are also important, and examine such features as the duration of the problem, and the likelihood of recovery or relapse (Von Korff 1992). The prognosis of a pain condition takes into consideration the risks of the condition progressing or remitting (Von Korff 1992).

Relative risk factors

An examination of relative risks will consider factors which contribute to the development of a pain problem, such as vibration or heavy manual work. For example, the Boeing group conducted a large prospective study of risks associated with acute industrial back problems (Bigos et al 1990). It was found that the most important risk factors were a previous history of back problems, low job satisfaction, and distress on the Minnesota Multiphasic Personality Inventory. Other possible risk factors included low endurance and smoking.

EXTENT OF THE PAIN PROBLEM

The epidemiological reports available may be considered according to the country of origin, the type of pain, or the type of sampling strategy. I will consider the available studies in terms of the country of origin (after all, we all like to think of a problem in terms of how it really affects us in *our* community). The bulk of the studies come from the USA and Canada, with others coming from New Zealand, Scandinavia and Great Britain.

Australia

No comprehensive, definitive epidemiological study of chronic pain in Australia has yet been published. In a report on the management of severe pain in Australia, the National Health and Medical Research Council (1988) called for the design and implementation of comprehensive epidemiological studies into chronic non-cancer pain. Such studies have not been forthcoming. Gross (1986) presented a preliminary report on a study of pain commissioned by the Australian Pain Society. The cost of chronic pain to the Australian community was put at $7.8 billion annually. Unfortunately, no further reports on this study are available.

Canada

Pain prevalence

A number of studies have examined pain in Canada. Of particular note is the ongoing work of Crook and her colleagues (1984, 1986, 1989). Beginning with a 1984 report, this group conducted an analytic telephone survey of 500 households which were randomly selected from the roster of a group family practice facility. The aim of the study was to determine the prevalence of pain and persistent pain in a community sample. A total of 394 households consented to participate in the survey, designed for people over the age of 18 years. A pain prevalence rate of 16% was found, with the rate of persistent pain being 11% for this community sample.

Persistent pain

In 1986, Crook et al compared the data from the 1984 community survey with data from a pain clinic sample of 62 patients. Not surprisingly, in contrast to the 11% report of persistent pain in the community sample, the pain clinic sample had an 86% report of persistent pain. A 2-year follow-up of both samples revealed that 46% of the family practice sample no longer had pain, while only 18% of the pain clinic sample no longer had pain (Crook et al 1989). We will return to these interesting findings again when we consider the natural history of pain.

Spinal disorders

Spitzer and his colleagues (1987) set out to determine the frequency of spinal disorders using the incidence rate from Workers Compensation files for the state of Quebec. They found that 1.69% of the total employed population was compensated at least once for a work-acquired spinal disorder in 1981. The actual incidence rate of spinal disorders which required a work absence was 1.37%, while the incidence rate for spinal disorders without an absence from work was 0.32%. The total cost of compensation claims for spinal disorders in Quebec in 1981 was $150 million. It was found that of all compensated claims for spinal disorders, the 7.4% which resulted in an absence from work of longer than 6 months accounted for 75.6% of all compensation costs.

Great Britain

Croft et al (1993) conducted a large cross-sectional population survey in the United Kingdom, drawing on the registered populations of two general practices. A questionnaire with a 1-month follow-up to non-responders was posted out to an age stratified random sample of 2034 people aged 18–25 years. Results showed that 56% of subjects reported having pain in the last month, 35% reported having chronic pain, and 13% reported having chronic widespread pain.

New Zealand

Work-related back pain

Burry and Gravis (1988) completed a survey of work-related back pain injury claimants reported during a 3-month period in 1984. The 420 claimants were men younger than 60 years of age. Rather than investigating prevalence, Burry and Gravis were interested in how such injuries occurred, whether they could have been prevented, and what was the outcome. They found that labourers, freezing workers, coal miners and railway workers had a high risk of injury. Lifting was the most common cause of injury, with over half of the cases involving a sudden strain. Encouragingly, 82% of claimants had returned to work within a 4-week period.

Back pain in nurses

Coggan and her colleagues (1994) completed a postal cross-sectional survey of all nurses employed by the Auckland Area Health Board in 1992 to examine the prevalence of back pain among nurses. A response rate of 82.7% was obtained for the survey, representing 4636 nurses. Results indicated that the lifetime prevalence of nursing-related back pain was 62.3%, with an annual prevalence of 36.8% and a point prevalence rate of 11.6%. The lifetime prevalence of back pain was 74.4%.

Common pains

Another large epidemiological study from New Zealand was conducted by James and her colleagues (1991). A probability sample of 1498 adults aged 18–64 years was obtained as part of the 1986 Christchurch Psychiatric Epidemiology Study. The Diagnostic Interview Schedule, which asks 11 questions about pain, was used in the study. Findings showed that 81.7% of subjects reported a pain experience, which was most commonly joint or back pain or headache.

Low back pain

Laslett et al (1991) undertook a telephone survey of 314 randomly selected urban New Zealanders to examine the extent of low back pain. A lifetime prevalence rate of 78.3% was found, along with an annual incidence rate of 30.7% and a point incidence rate of 17.8%. In 63.2% of cases, the first episode of low back pain occurred before the age of 30 years. In 33.3% of the sample, the pain was reported as being chronic rather than acute. The researchers found no correlation between the frequency of pain and the occupational postures of the subjects.

Scandinavia

Persistent pain

Andersson and his group (1993) in Sweden examined pain in a randomly selected sample of 15% (n = 1806) of the population of two Swedish primary health care districts. A response rate of 90% was obtained, with subjects aged 25–74 years. Findings indicated that 55% of subjects had persistent pain lasting for more than 3 months, while 49% had persistent pain of longer than 6 months duration. 90% of the subjects had pain which was musculoskeletal in origin. A further 12.8% were classified as having dysfunctional chronic pain. Chronic pain was highest among blue-collar workers and lowest among white-collar workers.

Pain in the general population

Pain in the general population in Sweden was also investigated by Brattberg et al (1989). Using a survey posted to 1009 randomly-selected adults between the ages of 18 and 84 years, 827 responses were received.

The findings were that 66% reported having pain, 40% had obvious pain, and 31.3% had back pain.

Rheumatic pain

A random sample of 900 individuals from a 1984 health survey in Sweden were invited to participate in a study (Jacobsson et al 1989) of the prevalence of rheumatic complaints of more than 6 weeks duration which had occurred in the previous year. A total of 445 people agreed to take part and were examined by a rheumatologist. A further 431 people were recruited by the rheumatologist, of whom only 89% were directly examined by the rheumatologist. A 37.8% overall prevalence rate for rheumatic diseases was found in the general population group.

Fibromyalgia

Makela and Heliovaara (1991) examined the prevalence of primary fibromyalgia in Finland using a cross-sectional survey of 8000 people 30 years of age or over. From 3434 people who attended a clinical examination, the prevalence of fibromyalgia was found to be only 0.75%. Its presence was related to female gender, occupation (no cases among white-collar workers), educational level (higher prevalence among those with lower education), work stress (higher in those with high levels of physical stress), and age (greatest in those aged 55–64 years).

Low back pain

Another Finnish study has examined the extent of health care services used by patients with low back pain in a population-based primary health care setting (Rekola et al 1993). Help for low back pain was required by 234 patients (3.5% of the sample). Just over half of these patients (51%) had additional visits to the health service due to musculoskeletal pain, but only 39% were due to further low back pain. The patients with musculoskeletal problems had twice the annual average number of visits to a primary health care practice than did those without musculoskeletal problems.

United States of America

Musculoskeletal problems

Cunningham and Kelsey (1984) examined the prevalence of musculoskeletal impairments in American adults using a stratified probability sample from the 1971–1975 United States Health and Nutrition Examination Survey (HANES). The study of 6913 people involved a medical examination combined with an interview. Findings revealed that 32.6% of participants had musculoskeletal symptoms as determined by a physician, while 29.7% reported having musculoskeletal symptoms. Back trouble was the most frequently seen complaint (15–17%), followed by knee problems (12–15%).

Chronic pain

The National Health and Nutrition Examination Survey (HANES I) for 1971–1975 was also used in an augmentation survey by Magni et al (1990). A complete data set was obtained on 3023 adults aged 25–74 years. It was found that 14.4% suffered from chronic pain, while 7.4% had some pain but were not sure if it was chronic. Medical treatment had been sought by 82.7% of the chronic pain group.

Back pain

Reisbord and Greenland (1985) completed a study of the self-report of back pain prevalence among a probability sample of 2792 adults in Ohio. They found that women had a 4% higher prevalence rate of back pain than did men, with the highest prevalence (44–66%) appearing in women aged 50–64 years who were no longer married. The lowest prevalence rates (9–11%) were found in married men with greater than high school education.

Nuprin pain report

The Nuprin Pain Report was the result of a national survey of 1254 people aged 18 years or over (Sternbach 1986a, 1986b). It is one of the most widely cited epidemiological studies of pain. The study found that the most commonly occurring pain complaints were headache (73%), followed by backaches (56%), muscle pains (53%) and joint pains (51%). It was also found that younger people experienced more pains than older people (except for joint pains), white persons had more pain than black or Hispanic persons, and that there were no major differences in the pain prevalences between households with different incomes.

Types of pain

A random stratified sample of members of a Group Health Cooperative aged 18–75 years participated in the study by Von Korff et al (1988). A mailed survey with a follow-up mailing plus a telephone follow-up was used to elicit 1016 responses. The prevalence of back pain in the previous

6 months was 41%, headache prevalence was 26%, abdominal pain 17%, chest pain 12%, and facial pain 12%. Recurrent persistent pain was found in 45% of the subjects, and severe and persistent pain was found in 8%. Cases of severe and persistent pain of 7 or more days in duration where activity was limited occurred in 2.7%, while severe, persistent pain, where activity was limited and three or more signs of pain dysfunction were found, occurred in 1.0% of the sample.

General reviews

Osterweis et al (1987), in a comprehensive review of the pain epidemiological literature, found that low back pain is the most common type of chronic pain, with other common pains being head pain, muscle pain, joint pain, dental pain, stomach pain and menstrual and pre-menstrual pain. They estimated that between 10% and 15% of workers will experience some work-related disability from back pain every year.

Goodman and McGrath (1991) have provided a comprehensive review of the epidemiological literature dealing with pain in children and adolescents. While pointing to a number of design and methodology problems in such studies, they reviewed over 50 studies which have looked at specific conditions such as abdominal pain, head pain, and pain in hospitalized patients. Although they concluded that much needs to be done to improve the epidemiological understanding of pain in children and adolescents, their review has provided some useful information which will be referred to in the section on children's pain in Chapter 8.

NATURAL HISTORY OF PAIN

Information on the natural history of non-cancer pain conditions is somewhat sparse. Most attention has been given to uncovering the natural history of back pain, and as Von Korff (1994) notes, data is 'incomplete and confusing'. Von Korff (1994) has suggested that back pain is typically of a recurrent nature. Most people who have an acute back pain episode do improve, but they may have future episodes of back pain, some of which may be chronic in nature. The findings of Rekola and his colleagues (1993) echo Von Korff's point: over half of their sample of patients with low back pain required further treatment for musculoskeletal pain problems.

The work of Crook et al (1986), which was reported earlier in this chapter, is also pertinent here. More of those patients being treated at pain clinic (82%) continued to have pain problems at a 2-year follow-up than did the family practice patients (54%). These findings suggest that it is those persons with more complicated pain problems who are seen at pain clinic. If the pain severity and complexity is greater to begin with, it is understandable that these problems may persist more. Additionally, it is important to note that some 54% of the family practice patients in the study by Crook et al (1986) continued to have pain problems. This is a similar figure to that reported by Rekola et al (1993).

AETIOLOGICAL FACTORS IN DEVELOPING CHRONIC PAIN

Aetiological factors are those which have been shown to have some relationship with an increased risk of developing pain (Bombardier et al 1994). Such factors may relate to the person's environment, their occupation, their behaviour, their lifestyle, their genetic makeup, or to demographic factors (Bombardier et al 1994). Most consideration of aetiological factors and pain has been given to the condition of back pain.

Back pain – risk factors

Frymoyer and his colleagues (1980) examined the records of 3920 patients who were seen over a 3-year period at an American family practice clinic. After finding that 11% of men and 9% of women had experienced an episode of low back pain, they then examined the contribution of possible risk factors. The study considered both occupational risk factors and the non-occupational risk factors of driving history, sporting history, smoking and pregnancy history. Patients of both sexes with back pain were found to perform significantly more lifting, carrying, pulling, pushing, bending and twisting at work, were exposed to more stressful events, had greater anxiety and depression, and were more likely to be smokers with a chronic cough, than were people without back pain. More older men than younger men had back pain, and more of those with pain were truckdrivers. Women with back pain had had more pregnancies than women without back pain.

Biering-Sørensen (1984) found that good isometric back-muscle endurance had a protective role in preventing the first occurrence of low back trouble, while weak trunk muscles and the reduced flexibility of the back and hamstrings were more frequent in those who had recurring back problems.

In examining the relationship between low back pain and work factors among 1760 women, Svensson and Andersson (1989) found that forward bending, lifting, standing, monotonous work, dissatisfaction with work tasks and the work environment, worry and fatigue at the end of the day were all significantly related to the occurrence of low back pain. When the correlations between variables were taken into account, only the variables of dissatisfaction with work and increased worry and fatigue at the end of the day were significantly correlated with low back pain occurrence.

> **Box 2.1** Risk factors in the development of work-related low back pain. The most frequently mentioned risk factors (Bombardier et al 1994) are:
>
> - younger age
> - male sex
> - heavy physical work
> - manual handling
> - non-neutral trunk postures
> - whole body vibration
> - an earlier incident of back pain
> - a low level of fitness
> - low trunk strength
> - low job satisfaction
> - work monotony
> - smoking.

Bombardier et al (1994) have provided a summary of frequently mentioned risk factors in the development of work-related low back pain and these are given in Box 2.1.

SUMMARY OF EPIDEMIOLOGICAL FINDINGS

The epidemiological studies from a number of countries tell us that the incidence of pain in the general community is noteworthy, with study estimates ranging from 16% to 81.7%: Crook et al (1984) found an incidence rate of 16%; Cunningham and Kelsey (1984) found an incidence rate of 32.6%; Jacobsson et al (1989) found an incidence rate of 37.8%; Croft et al (1993) found an incidence rate of 56%; Brattberg et al (1989) found an incidence rate of 66%; while James et al (1991) found an incidence rate of 81.7%.

The estimates for the incidence of persistent/recurrent/chronic pain show less variance, with the range being 11% to 55%: Crook et al (1984) reported the figure as 11%; Magni et al (1990) reported this incidence as 14.4%; Von Korff et al (1990) reported a 45% incidence; while Andersson et al (1993) found a 55% incidence rate for persistent pain of longer than 3 months duration.

In terms of the types of pains which worry members of the community, problems are clearly experienced with back pain, musculoskeletal pain (including muscle and joint pains), headache, and stomach pains.

With respect to the natural history of pain problems, in most cases of acute pain, the pain will abate, and individuals will resume their normal occupational activities. However, such individuals seem to be more likely to have further episodes of pain problems, and these do not necessarily arise in the same body part. In about 50% of cases, pain will recur.

If we look at back pain in particular, it has been estimated that 70–80%

of the population will suffer from a back disorder at some time during their lives (Addison 1985, Deyo 1988, NOH&SC 1989). Some 10% of these people will go on to develop a chronic pain disorder. 10–15% of adults will have some degree of work disability due to back pain each year (Osterweis et al 1987).

Approximately 20% of all work injuries involve the spinal column (Spitzer et al 1987). Spinal/back pain has been called 'the most common chronic pain' (Osterweis et al 1987). Spitzer et al (1987) found that 1.69% of the employed population was compensated at least once for a spinal disorder acquired at work. In the United States of America, low back pain has been described as 'the most expensive benign condition in America' (Mayer et al 1987).

The frequency of back-pain-related work disability has increased over time (Osterweis et al 1987). Frymoyer (1993) reported that low back disorders resulting in disability have been increasing at a greater rate than any other health problem. Yet he points out that the epidemiological literature shows that there is little variance in the annual incidence rate of low back problems. As Deyo (1993) said, 'Current methods of management are not preventing an epidemic of low back pain'.

Linton (1987) and Schug and Large (1993) have put the case for the prevention of chronic pain conditions due to the difficulties in resolving problems for people with chronic pain. Prevention of injury, and better early management of pain conditions will play an important part in the prevention of chronic pain. 'Because occupational activities contribute substantially to the development and course of low back pain, modification of factors in the work site is an important approach to the prevention of low back pain' (Kelsey et al 1990).

IMPLICATIONS FOR OCCUPATIONAL THERAPISTS

An examination of the literature suggests that pain is a common problem in our communities. Given its extent, it is important for all health professionals, including occupational therapists, to be aware of the needs of patients with various types of pain, and to have knowledge of the different approaches that can be adopted for managing both acute and chronic pain. Health professionals also need to recognize the importance of preventive management in minimizing the original and recurrent pain episodes.

The role of the occupational therapist in preventive occupational health and safety programs cannot be overemphasized – it makes good sense to close the stable door *before* the horse has bolted. Similarly, it is sound practice to prevent the occurrence of injuries which might result in ongoing pain problems. In looking at prevention programs, it becomes clear from the literature on aetiological factors that consideration needs to be given not only to the physical factors in the environment (for example, bench heights and lifting load limits), but also to factors such as task variety and opportunities for challenge. Of course, worker characteristics (for example, the degree of physical fitness) and behaviours (for example, correct body mechanics) are also important.

In the next chapter, a detailed account will be given of the various models of pain management. Given its importance, back pain will be considered in some detail. Once familiar with the overarching management models for pain, the occupational therapist can then look to the particular occupational therapy orientations useful in working with individuals with pain.

CHAPTER SUMMARY

Examination of the data from the United States of America, New Zealand, Australia, Sweden, Finland, Great Britain and Canada provides support for the widespread experience of acute and chronic pain in our communities. We can say with some confidence that pain is quite prevalent in the community, and that the incidence of chronic pain ranges from 16-82%, with around 50% of chronic pain being due to low back problems. The cost of chronic pain in general is enormous, and chronic back pain in particular is a major problem.

Looking at acute pain states, the majority of cases will quickly resolve with only around 10% going on to develop chronic conditions. Currently, we are unable to make definitive statements on the natural history of the chronic pain phenomenon. While the work of Crook and her colleagues (1984, 1986, 1989) suggests that a percentage of both treated and untreated people with chronic pain will improve over time, perhaps half have recurring pain problems. In other words, some chronic pain conditions resolve, and some do not. Furthermore, the risk of repeated injury and pain seems greater for those who have already had a pain incident. Occupational therapists have a responsibility to assist in the prevention of pain problems, the prevention of further injury and pain, and in the management of those individuals with ongoing chronic pain problems.

REFERENCES

Addison R G 1985 Chronic low back pain (CLO-BAP). The Clinical Journal of Pain 1: 50–59
Andersson H I, Ejlertsson G, Leden I, Rosenberg C 1993 Chronic pain in a geographically defined general population: studies of differences in age, gender, social class, and pain localization. Clinical Journal of Pain 9: 174–182
Biering-Sørensen F 1984 Physical measurements as risk indicators for low-back trouble over a one-year period. Spine 9: 106–119

Bigos S J, Battie M C, Nordin M, Spengler D M, Guy D P 1990 Industrial back injury. In: Weinstein J N, Wiesel W (eds) The lumbar spine. The International Association for the Study of the Lumbar Spine, Saunders, Philadelphia

Bombardier C, Kerr M S, Shannon H S, Frank J W 1994 A guide to interpreting epidemiologic studies on the etiology of back pain. Spine 19(18): 2047S–2056S

Brattberg G, Thorslund M, Wikman A 1989 The prevalence of pain in a general population: the results of a postal survey in a county of Sweden. Pain 37: 215–222

Burry H C, Gravis V 1988 Compensated back injury in New Zealand. New Zealand Medical Journal 101: 542–544

Coggan C, Norton R, Roberts I, Hope V 1994 Prevalence of back pain among nurses. New Zealand Medical Journal 107: 306–308

Croft P, Rigby A S, Boswell R, Schollum J, Silman A 1993 The prevalence of chronic widespread pain in the general population. Journal of Rheumatology 20: 710–713

Crombie I K, Davies H T O, Macrae W A 1994 The epidemiology of chronic pain: time for new directions. Pain 57: 1–3

Crook J, Rideout E, Browne G 1984 The prevalence of pain complaints in a general population. Pain 18: 299–314

Crook J, Tunks E, Rideout E, Browne G 1986 Epidemiological comparison of persistent pain sufferers in a specialty pain clinic and in the community. Archives of Physical Medicine and Rehabilitation 76: 451–455

Crook J, Weir R, Tunks E 1989 An epidemiological follow-up survey of persistent pain sufferers in a group family practice and specialty pain clinic. Pain 36: 49–61

Cunningham L S, Kelsey J L 1984 Epidemiology of musculoskeletal impairments and associated disability. American Journal of Public Health 74: 574–579

Deyo R A 1988 Measuring the functional status of patients with low back pain. Archives of Physical Medicine and Rehabilitation 69: 1044–1053

Deyo R A 1993 Practice variations, treatment fads, rising disability: do we need a new clinical research paradigm? Spine 18: 2153–2162

Frymoyer J W 1993 Quality: an international challenge to the diagnosis and treatment of disorders of the lumbar spine. Spine 18: 2147–2152

Frymoyer J W, Pope M H, Costanza M C, Rosen J C, Goggin J E, Wilder D G 1980 Epidemiologic studies of low-back pain. Spine 5: 419–423

Goodman J E, McGrath P J 1991 The epidemiology of pain in children and adolescents: a review. Pain 46: 247–264

Gross P 1986 The economic costs of chronic pain in Australia. Proceedings of the 8th Annual Scientific Meeting of the Australian Pain Society, Melbourne, Australia

Jacobsson L, Lindgarde F, Manthorpe R 1989 The commonest rheumatic complaints of over six weeks' duration in a twelve-month period in a defined Swedish population. Scandinavian Journal of Rheumatology 18: 353–360

James F R, Large R G, Bushnell J A, Wells J E 1991 Epidemiology of pain in New Zealand. Pain 44: 279–283

Kelsey J L, Golden A L, Mundt D J 1990 Low back pain/prolapsed lumbar intervertebral disc. Rheumatic Disease Clinics of North America 16: 699–716

Laslett M, Crothers C, Beattie P, Cregten L, Moses A 1991 The frequency and incidence of low back pain/sciatica in an urban population. New Zealand Medical Journal 104: 424–426

Linton S J 1987 Chronic pain: the case for prevention. Behaviour Research and Therapy 25: 313–317

Lowe C R, Kostrzewski J 1973 Epidemiology: a guide to teaching methods. Churchill Livingstone, Edinburgh

Magni G, Caldieron C, Rigatti-Luchini S, Merskey H 1990 Chronic musculoskeletal pain and depressive symptoms in the general population: an analysis of the 1st National Health and Nutrition Examination Survey data. Pain 43: 299–307

Makela M, Heliovaara M 1991 Prevalence of primary fibromyalgia in the Finnish population. British Medical Journal 303: 216–219

Mayer T G, Gatchel R J, Mayer H, Kishino N D, Keeley J, Mooney V 1987 A prospective two-year study of functional restoration in industrial low back injury. JAMA 258: 1763–1767

Merskey H (ed) 1986 Classification of chronic pain: description of chronic pain syndromes and definitions of pain terms. Pain 24(3): S217

National Health and Medical Research Council 1988 Management of severe pain: report of the working party on management of severe pain. Australian Government Publishing Service, Canberra

National Occupational Health and Safety Commission 1989 National strategy for the prevention of occupational back pain. Australian Government Publishing Service, Canberra

Osterweis M, Kleinman A, Mechanic D 1987 Pain and disability: clinical, behavioral, and public policy perspectives. National Academy Press, Washington DC

Reisbord L S, Greenland S 1985 Factors associated with self reported back-pain prevalence: a population-based study. Journal of Chronic Diseases 38: 691–702

Rekola K E, Keinanen-Kiukaanniemi S, Takals J 1993 Use of health services by patients seeking care for low back symptoms: a population-based prospective study of consultations with primary care physicians. Journal of Musculoskeletal Medicine 1: 55–64

Schug S A, Large R G 1993 Economic considerations in pain management. PharmacoEconomics 3: 260–267

Spitzer W O, LeBlanc F E, Dupuis M et al 1987 Scientific approach to the assessment and management of activity-related spinal disorders: a monograph for clinicians. Report of the Quebec Task Force on Spinal Disorders. Spine Supplement 12: S1–S55

Sternbach R A 1986a Survey of pain in the United States: the Nuprin Pain Report. Clinical Journal of Pain 2: 49–53

Sternbach R A 1986b Pain and 'hassles' in the United States: findings of the Nuprin Pain Report. Pain 27: 69–80

Svensson H O, Andersson G B J 1989 The relationship of low-back pain, work history, work environment and stress. Spine 14: 517–522

Von Korff M 1992 Epidemiological and survey methods: chronic pain assessment. In: Turk D C, Melzack R (eds) Handbook of pain assessment. Guilford, New York

Von Korff M 1994 Studying the natural history of back pain. Spine 19(18): 2041S–2046S

Von Korff M, Dworkin S F, Le Resche L, Kruger A 1988 An epidemiological comparison of pain complaints. Pain 32: 173–183

Von Korff M, Dworkin S F, Le Resche L 1990 Graded chronic pain status: an epidemiological evaluation. Pain 40: 279–291

3

Models for intervention

Development of the multidisciplinary
  approach 29
Definition of terms 30
Acute pain management models 31
Chronic pain management
  models 31
Chronic cancer pain management 32
Chronic non-cancer pain
  management 33
  Aims 33

Treatment approaches 33
Efficacy of multidisciplinary pain
  management programs 36
Early intervention and prevention
  programs 36
  Primary prevention approach 37
  Secondary prevention approach 37
Chapter summary 38
References 39

In Chapters 1 and 2, allusion was made to the fact that different management models are used to treat pain of different types. In this chapter, we examine in more detail current management models for acute pain and chronic pain, chronic cancer pain and chronic non-cancer pain and prevention programs. But first, we look briefly at the development of the multidisciplinary approach which has revolutionized modern pain management.

DEVELOPMENT OF THE MULTIDISCIPLINARY APPROACH

When someone has pain in normal circumstances (we exclude here exceptional circumstances such as wars and sporting challenges like marathon races and football matches), it is natural to seek the alleviation of that pain, and to worry that it may signal something sinister happening to one's body. If I were to develop pain at this moment, then my first course of action might be to take a mild analgesic. If the pain remained, then my next action would be to go to my doctor so that she could investigate its causes and take the pain away. Now, if my visit to the doctor did not result in the elimination of my pain, I would probably try another doctor who could take my pain away.

Such an approach is often effective for acute pain problems, but it is not effective for the many chronic pain conditions which afflict humankind. Until the 1960s and 1970s, this sequential doctor-attending was the common management method for patients with chronic pain, and treatment approaches were aimed at the symptomatic relief of chronic pain (Cairns et al 1976). However, such conventional medical approaches were not effective in treating the patient with the chronic pain syndrome (Hartman & Ainsworth 1980, Keefe 1982, Turner 1982).

The founder of the multidisciplinary approach for the management of chronic pain was Dr J J Bonica (Melzack & Wall 1983). He realized that complex pain problems required the knowledge and experience of a variety of specialists working together in a multidisciplinary or interdisciplinary team (Bonica 1984). Having experts from different disciplines assess the patient and come together to arrive at a diagnosis and develop an integrated management plan seemed to him to be far preferable to the existing approach of sequential examination by multiple experts who diagnosed and treated in isolation, and then sent the patient on to the next specialist when they could not find a cure. Thus, the multidisciplinary or interdisciplinary pain clinic for the assessment and management of patients with chronic pain conditions was born (Bonica 1984, Carlson 1979, Hallett & Pilowsky 1982).

While the literature talks of an interdisciplinary pain clinic or a multidisciplinary pain clinic, it has been my experience that most pain clinics use the latter approach. A multidisciplinary approach is one where a number of experts from different disciplines assess the patient and report back to the team coordinator (who is usually a medical practitioner), who then coordinates the decision making and program planning, whereas an interdisciplinary approach involves those same professionals coming together after assessing the patient, and coming to a consensus on program planning (Jacobs et al 1989).

DEFINITION OF TERMS

Box 3.1 gives the International Association for the Study of Pain's definitions of terms describing pain management facilities (Loeser 1991).

Box 3.1 IASP definitions of pain management facilities

Pain treatment facility. Any type of facility which treats pain problems, regardless of the type of professional involvement or the type of patient seen.
Multidisciplinary pain centre. A multidisciplinary group of health professionals and scientists with the roles of patient care, teaching and research for acute and chronic pain problems.
Multidisciplinary pain clinic. A multidisciplinary health delivery facility with the role of managing patients with chronic pain.
Pain clinic. A facility, lacking interdisciplinary assessment and management, which is concerned with the management of patients with chronic pain.
Modality-oriented clinic. A facility which provides a specific type of treatment rather than a comprehensive assessment and management program (Loeser 1991).

While these terms are defined for clarity, it should be pointed out that the term 'pain clinic' has been used as a generic one in much of the literature. In this book, in keeping with this tradition, I have used the term 'pain clinic' to refer to a multidisciplinary or interdisciplinary pain management program with a mix of medical and allied health practitioners.

ACUTE PAIN MANAGEMENT MODELS

In the past, acute pain management was regarded as a simple practice. It was the sort of thing which had been working well, or so we thought. Acute pain is a consequence of some injury, or illness or trauma, or is a consequence of surgical procedures. Postoperative pain is one of the main causes of acute pain (Schug & Large 1993). As such, acute pain should be easily managed by appropriate analgesia and adjuvant therapies.

However, it came as a shock to some to find (in the 1980s) that much acute pain was being poorly managed, particularly postoperative pain (Cohen 1980, Cousins 1991, Cousins & Mather 1989). Cousins (1991) observed that postoperative pain is treated effectively in less than 30–50% of patients! Similarly, in a survey of 454 patients in hospital medical and surgical wards, it was found that 60% had pain of moderate to severe intensity (Donovan et al 1987). One problem with acute pain management lay with the frequent use of intramuscular opioids given 'as required'. The concerns of medical and nursing staff that the patient would become addicted, combined with the concerns of the patient that he was being a nuisance, all acted against effective pain relief.

In recent years, a more proactive, concerted approach has been taken to acute pain management, with the use of such techniques as pre-emptive analgesia (prior to surgery), patient-controlled analgesia and continuous regional anaesthesia (Schug & Large 1993). For a comprehensive review of the state of the art of acute pain management, the reader is referred to Cousins (1989, 1991) and Woolf (1989).

The role of the occupational therapist

With respect to the role of the occupational therapist in acute pain management, the key areas of contribution here relate to areas of hand therapy, burn management and adversive procedural pain in children. More comprehensive coverage of the occupational therapy role will be given in Chapter 8.

CHRONIC PAIN MANAGEMENT MODELS

Until recently, a clear distinction has been made between the management of chronic pain of cancer origin versus chronic pain of non-cancer origin.

Much controversy currently exists in the pain world about the use of opioids for chronic non-cancer pain. For example, Portenoy and Foley (1986) suggested that opioids could be used safely with patients with non-malignant pain. On the other hand, Large and Schug (1995) have cautioned against the use of opioids for individuals with chronic pain of non-cancer origin.

In this book, rather than restate the arguments for the use of one or another of these approaches, I will adopt the, until recently, widely accepted convention of distinct management approaches for cancer pain and non-cancer pain. The reader is referred to the recent papers by Large and Schug (1995) and Somerville (1995) for an interesting and up-to-date overview of the opioid controversy.

CHRONIC CANCER PAIN MANAGEMENT

The mainstay of the management of the patient with chronic pain of cancer origin has been the use of a wide array of pharmacological agents, combined with appropriate surgical interventions, radiotherapeutic methods, chemotherapy and hormone therapy (Stuart & Cramond 1993). The goal of therapy is the alleviation of pain, support for the patient and the patient's family, the control of distressing symptoms, lifestyle adjustment and anticancer therapy (Cramond & Stuart 1993). The overall aim is to provide pain relief, and when malignancy is far advanced, to help the patient to enjoy their remaining time as pain free as possible and to die with dignity (Sternbach 1974).

WHO analgesic ladder

The World Health Organization has developed an analgesic ladder which recommends a 3-step method for alleviating cancer pain. The first step on the ladder begins with the use of non-opioid drugs with or without adjuvant therapies. The medications of choice here are aspirin and the non-steroidal anti-inflammatory preparations. If the pain continues, then step 2 of the ladder suggests the addition of a weak opioid medication such as codeine. If the pain still persists or gets worse, then step 3 of the ladder recommends the use of a strong opioid like morphine.

Surgical interventions

In cases of advanced malignancy where larger and larger doses of opioids are required for pain relief, resulting in a clouding of consciousness or where activity-related pain cannot be controlled, neurosurgical techniques such as percutaneous cervical cordotomies and ventriculostomies may be indicated. Percutaneous cervical cordotomy is a useful technique for patients who experience unilateral cancer pain below the head and neck

(Stuart & Cramond 1993). The procedure involves a lesion being made in the spinothalamic tract at Cl–C2 (Stuart & Cramond 1993). For those patients with pain from cancer of the head or neck, or bilateral, midline or diffuse cancer pain, a ventriculostomy may be helpful. This involves the insertion of a morphine reservoir into the lateral cerebral ventricle (Cramond & Stuart 1993). Such patients can then be given good pain relief with very small doses of morphine.

The role of the occupational therapist

With respect to the role which the occupational therapist plays in the management of patients with cancer pain, Cramond and Stuart (1993) reported that the occupational therapist assists with the home safety of the patient after ventriculostomy. A more complete coverage of the management of cancer pain and the occupational therapy contribution will be given in the special topics section of this book (Ch. 8).

CHRONIC NON-CANCER PAIN MANAGEMENT

The goal of management for patients with chronic pain of non-cancer origin is 'to rehabilitate the patient to an improved quality of life independently of achieved reduction of the experience of pain' (Arner 1983).

As outlined earlier, the major treatment facility developed to manage patients with chronic non-cancer pain is the multidisciplinary pain clinic. Pain clinics vary from centre to centre in the treatment approach used, the population catered for and the type of professional personnel involved (Hallett & Pilowsky 1982, Roberts 1983). The treatment approach adopted is dependent upon how chronic pain is conceptualized (Roy 1984).

Aims

A number of aims are common across pain clinics. These aims are to improve the patient's level of functioning (Roy 1984, Strong 1989), to enhance the quality and productivity of the patient's life (Little 1981, Arner 1983), to reduce or eliminate pain if possible (Katz 1983), to control pain behaviour through behavioural and self-help techniques (Roy 1984), to gather and exchange information which might be lost in separate clinics (Roy 1984), to educate other staff about pain management (Katz 1983, Roberts 1983), and to promote research into aspects of chronic pain (Katz 1983, Roberts 1983).

Treatment approaches

Treatment approaches used with patients with chronic non-cancer pain also vary according to the type of guiding theoretical conceptualization of chronic pain ascribed to by the facility personnel. The predominant philosophies include the operant behavioural approach, the cognitive behavioural approach, an eclectic rehabilitation or multimodal approach, a sports medicine approach, and a functional restoration approach. The main components of these different approaches are briefly reviewed below.

Operant behavioural

Operant behavioural approaches are concerned with modifying 'excess disability and expressions of suffering' (Fordyce et al 1985). Operant behavioural techniques are concerned with the modification of a person's pain behaviours rather than their nociception (or pain) itself. Pain behaviours refer to those overt expressions that one is in pain. They may include such things as grimacing, moaning, bracing oneself, guarding particular body parts, and using various supports such as walking sticks, neck collars, arm splints and wheelchairs.

The goals of operant approaches usually include (Turk & Rudy 1990):

- a reduction in pain behaviours
- a reduction in the use of medication
- a reduction in the use of health care resources
- an increase in the person's activity levels
- the restoration of well behaviours
- the modification of contingencies which reinforce both pain behaviours and well behaviours within the patient's environment.

Cognitive behavioural

Cognitive behavioural techniques, while embracing some of the features of the operant behavioural approach, acknowledge the importance of a person's thoughts and beliefs, that is, their cognitions, about the pain problem. Professor Dennis Turk has been the champion of the cognitive behavioural approach to pain management.

The goals of a cognitive behavioural approach often include (Turk & Rudy 1988):

- modifying the patient's view of his problems, enabling him to see them as manageable rather than overwhelming
- convincing the patient that he can learn the skills he needs to cope
- changing the patient's view of himself from passive, reactive and helpless to active, resourceful and competent
- equipping the patient with the skills to monitor thoughts, feelings and behaviours and to learn the interrelationships between these

- teaching the patient how and when to use the necessary behaviours required for adaptive response to his problems
- encouraging the patient to attribute success to his own efforts
- helping the patient to anticipate problems which may arise and preparing ways to deal with them.

Eclectic rehabilitation or multimodal

Many pain management programs do not subscribe exclusively to one management approach, choosing instead to incorporate parts of particular approaches such as the cognitive behavioural approach. Such non-exclusive approaches can be labelled eclectic or multimodal. Eclectic rehabilitation or multimodal approaches inevitably involve the combined application of a number of techniques which usually include:

- the use of supportive medication, with set rather than on-demand schedules
- education about pain
- group or individual psychotherapy
- relaxation training
- physiotherapy techniques such as transcutaneous nerve stimulation (TCNS) and exercise
- occupational therapy techniques such as occupational role assessment and task adaptation.

Such multimodal programs have been defined as ones in which various disciplines cooperate and which contain various treatment techniques (Corry et al 1992).

The goals of such approaches, though not well documented and variable across centres, appear to be to modify nociception to a degree (through the application of such things as TCNS, supportive medication and relaxation) to enable the patient to resume relevant life roles. Corry and his colleagues (1992) state that '...the aim of such programmes was described as teaching patients better ways of living with this pain or coping with the pain'.

Sports medicine

The sports medicine approach to chronic pain management is a somewhat newer approach. This approach utilizes a more proactive, aggressive intervention which is ideally begun earlier, before too many additional complications of chronicity set in. Like the behavioural approach, the goal of the sports medicine approach is not to modify nociception. Increasing fitness levels is a major goal, as is resumption of previous life roles. The working through pain philosophy is common. The slogan 'no pain, no gain' is an apt one here.

Functional restoration

The functional restoration approach has been advocated by Mayer and his colleagues (1987). The goals of this approach are to:

- quantify the status of the patient using physical function tests and patient self-report
- physically recondition the injured functional units of the patients
- engage the patients in work simulation and whole body retraining
- engage the patients in a cognitive behavioural disability management program
- make ongoing outcome assessment using objective criteria.

Efficacy of multidisciplinary pain management programs

Many studies have now been undertaken to evaluate the efficacy of multidisciplinary pain management programs (Turk & Rudy 1990). Most studies suggest that there is an initial improvement for many patients who participate in such programs (Turk & Rudy 1991) (for example, a colleague and I recently demonstrated an improvement in functioning for patients who participated in a back rehabilitation program (Moran & Strong 1995). However, a relapse rate ranging from 30–70% can be seen at follow-up (Turk & Rudy 1991). Clearly, further attention needs to be directed towards the long-term maintenance of gains from multidisciplinary pain programs.

The role of the occupational therapist

Occupational therapists are very often core members of the multi-disciplinary team working with patients with chronic non-cancer pain. The specific occupational therapy role in this important pain management area is dealt with further in Chapters 4, 6 and 7.

EARLY INTERVENTION AND PREVENTION PROGRAMS

Given the enormous burden incurred due to chronic pain problems, it would be sensible to devote more attention to prevention. Indeed, many workers have called for a concerted effort to be directed towards prevention programs and the call has been heeded at many levels, ranging from early and better management of acute pain to prevent chronicity (Schug & Large 1993), to legislative reforms for better workplace health and safety regulations and early rehabilitation. Prevention programs need to include both primary prevention to prevent initial injury and pain, and secondary prevention to prevent the recurrence of, and to reduce the severity of, pain problems (King 1993).

Primary prevention approach

Given that low back pain is a disorder having a marked impact upon the workplace (see, for example, Spitzer et al 1987), it is understandable and commendable that efforts have been directed towards the prevention of back injuries in the workplace. One such method is the back school approach (King 1993). Back school prevention programs focus on both the individual worker and the management (King 1993). Through education about the risk factors contributing to back pain, workers are encouraged to take responsibility for their own health and well-being and, concurrently, management are encouraged to develop early injury detection systems and early management systems, whereby someone with an injury can continue in the workplace in a modified job (King 1993).

King (1993), in reviewing the efficacy of back schools in the prevention of back injuries, found a number of methodological problems related to the use of different outcome variables, teaching methods, topics addressed and program participants. A major problem was the lack of controlled and randomized trials. Such methodological shortcomings are not confined to prevention program outcome: they have plagued all areas of pain management outcome studies. Despite such limitations, King (1993) commented that 'primary prevention programs translated into financial savings and decreased incidence of LBP [low back pain]'.

Donaldson and his colleagues (1993) conducted a controlled randomized crossover trial of a back and neck pain prevention program at a Canadian health facility. The subjects in the control group were offered the education program after being in the control group for 3 months. All subjects were measured on the variables of pain intensity, back care knowledge, and surface EMG levels of the cervical and lumbar paraspinal muscles. Data was also collected on the number of back injuries, days lost and costs incurred by the facility over a 12-month period. The treatment intervention developed and implemented consisted of a 90-minute education class supplemented by an education booklet. Results of the study showed that the experimental subjects increased their knowledge of back care and reported less pain than did the controls, while the facility experienced a reduction in the costs associated with back injuries over a 12-month period.

Ulen and Armstrong (1992) have outlined a useful procedure to follow in the workplace which can identify risk factors of specific jobs. Based on job analysis of specific jobs, the approach then implements change to the particular workstation to reduce the identified ergonomic stressors.

Secondary prevention approach

In Chapter 2, it was pointed out that individuals who incur a back pain problem are at risk of further pain incidents. An occupational group with a high documented occurrence of back problems is that of nurses (Coggan et al 1994). Linton and his colleagues (1989, 1992) developed a secondary prevention program for nurses who were at risk of developing a chronic pain disorder. An intensive 5 days per week, 8 hours per day program which extended for 5 weeks was developed. The program utilized a combined physical therapy and behaviour therapy approach. Subjects were engaged in exercises for 4 hours per day, were given instruction in back care and ergonomics, learnt about pain control through relaxation and coping strategies, were instructed in lifestyle management including goal setting and problem solving, were helped to analyse situations of risk, and were guided in implementing these techniques through weekend homework practice. The efficacy of this intensive program was then examined by randomly assigning at-risk nurses to either a waiting list control group or the intervention program. A total of 66 nurses participated in the study. It was found that nurses in the experimental group showed significant improvements compared with the waiting list controls on all subjective variables (pain intensity, anxiety, fatigue, depression, sleep quality, helplessness and global marital satisfaction), and on pain behaviours. A follow-up of the 36 nurses from the experimental group performed 18 months post-program indicated that these nurses continued to have less pain, less fatigue, less helplessness, less depression, were more satisfied with their ability to perform activities of daily living, and used fewer medications than they did prior to the intervention (Linton & Bradley 1992).

The role of the occupational therapist

There is an important role for the occupational therapist in the area of both primary and secondary prevention programs. The occupational therapist is equipped with skills such as body mechanics knowledge, instruction techniques and task analysis, skills which are essential in both primary and secondary prevention programs. The occupational therapist's role in the work rehabilitation of the individual with pain will be covered further in Chapter 6.

CHAPTER SUMMARY

In this chapter, an overview has been given of the popular approaches to pain management in the areas of acute pain management, chronic cancer pain management, chronic non-cancer pain management, and pain prevention. The specific role of the occupational therapist in each of these approaches was mentioned briefly. Before discussing this role in greater detail, the next chapter examines occupational therapy involvement with patients with pain, and elucidates the occupational therapy practice models which can guide occupational therapists working in the area.

REFERENCES

Arner S 1983 Pain clinic: present and future views. In: Kaukinen S, Rosenberg P H (eds) Abstracts Acta Anaesthesiologica Scandinavica 27(7): 47

Bonica J J 1984 Pain research and therapy: recent advances and future needs. In: Kruger L, Liebeskind J C (eds) Advances in pain research and therapy, vol. 6. Neural mechanisms of pain. Raven, New York

Cairns D, Thomas L, Mooney V, Pace J B 1976 A comprehensive treatment approach to chronic low back pain. Pain 2: 301–308

Carlson C A 1979 Pain – some concepts. Scandinavian Journal of Rehabilitation Medicine 11: 149–150

Coggan C, Norton R, Roberts I, Hope V 1994 Prevalence of back pain among nurses. New Zealand Medical Journal 107: 306–308

Cohen F L 1980 Postsurgical pain relief: status and nurses' medication choices. Pain 9: 265

Corry A, Linssen G, Spinhoven P 1992 Multimodal treatment programmes for chronic pain: a quantitative analysis of existing research data. Journal of Psychosomatic Research 36: 275–286

Cousins M J 1989 Acute and postoperative pain. In: Wall P D, Melzack R (eds) Textbook of pain, 2nd edn. Churchill Livingstone, London

Cousins M J 1991 Prevention of postoperative pain. In: Bond M R, Charlton J E, Woolf C J Proceedings of the VIth World Congress on Pain. Elsevier, Amsterdam

Cousins M J, Mather L E 1989 Relief of post-operative pain: advances awaiting application. Medical Journal of Australia 150: 354–355

Cramond T, Stuart G 1993 Intraventricular morphine for intractable pain of advanced cancer. Journal of Pain and Symptom Management 8: 465–472

Donaldson C S, Stanger L M, Donaldson M V, Cram J, Stubick D L 1993 A randomized crossover investigation of a back pain and disability prevention program: possible mechanisms for change. Journal of Occupational Rehabilitation 3: 83–94

Donovan M, Dillon P, McGuire L 1987 Incidence and characteristics of pain in a sample of medical–surgical inpatients. Pain 30: 69–78

Fordyce W E, Roberts A H, Sternbach R A 1985 The behavioral management of chronic pain: a response to critics. Pain 22: 113–125

Hallett E C, Pilowsky I 1982 The response to treatment in a multidisciplinary pain clinic. Pain 12: 365–374

Hartman L M, Ainsworth K D 1980 Self-regulation of chronic pain. Canadian Journal of Psychiatry 25: 38–43

Jacobs P, Crichton E, Visotina M 1989 Practical approaches to mental health care. Macmillan, Melbourne

Katz R L 1983 Principles and function of a multidisciplinary pain clinic. Acta Anaesthesiologica Scandinavica 27(78): 45

Keefe F J 1982 Behavioral assessment and treatment of chronic pain: current status and future directions. Journal of Consulting and Clinical Psychology 50: 896–911

King P M 1993 Back injury prevention programs: a critical review. Journal of Occupational Rehabilitation 3: 145–158

Large R G, Schug S A 1995 Opioids for chronic pain of non-malignant origin – caring or crippling. Health Care Analysis 3: 5–11

Linton S J, Bradley L A, Jensen I, Spangfort E, Sundell L 1989 The secondary prevention of low back pain: a controlled study with follow-up. Pain 36: 197–207

Linton S J, Bradley L A 1992 An 18-month follow-up of a secondary prevention program for back pain: help and hindrance factors related to outcome maintenance. Clinical Journal of Pain 8: 227–236

Little T F 1981 Chronic pain: modern concepts in management. Australian Family Physician 10: 265–270

Loeser J 1991 Desirable characteristics for pain treatment facilities: report of the IASP taskforce. In: Bond M R, Charlton J E, Woolf C J Proceedings of the VIth World Congress on Pain. Elsevier, Amsterdam

Mayer T G, Gatchel R J, Mayer H, Kishino N D, Keeley J, Mooney V 1987 A prospective two-year study of functional restoration in industrial low back injury. JAMA 258: 1763–1767

Melzack R, Wall P D 1983 The challenge of pain. Basic Books, New York
Moran M, Strong J 1995 Outcomes of a rehabilitation programme for patients with chronic back pain. British Journal of Occupational Therapy (accepted)
Portenoy R K, Foley K M 1986 Chronic use of opioid analgesics in non-malignant pain: report of 38 cases. Pain 25: 171–186
Roberts M T S 1983 Pain relief clinics. Patient Management 7: 25–32
Roy R 1984 Pain clinics: reassessment of objectives and outcomes. Archives of Physical Medicine and Rehabilitation 65: 448–451
Schug S A, Large R G 1993 Economic considerations in pain management. PharmacoEcomonics 3: 260–267
Somerville M A 1995 Opioids for chronic pain of non-malignant origin – coercion or consent? Health Care Analysis 3: 12–14
Spitzer W O, Leblanc F E, Dupuis M et al 1987 Scientific approach to the assessment and management of activity-related spinal disorders. A monograph for clinicians. Report of the Quebec Task Force on Spinal Disorders. Spine 12 (Supp.): S1–S55
Sternbach R A 1974 Pain patients: traits and treatment. Academic Press, New York
Strong J 1989 The occupational therapist's contribution to the management of chronic pain. Patient Management 13: 43–50
Stuart G, Cramond T 1993 Role of percutaneous cervical cordotomy for pain of malignant origin. Medical Journal of Australia 158: 667–670
Turk D C, Rudy T E 1988 A cognitive behavioral perspective on chronic pain: beyond the scalpel and syringe. In: Tollison C D (ed) Handbook of chronic pain management. Williams and Wilkins, Baltimore
Turk D C, Rudy T E 1990 Neglected factors in chronic pain treatment outcome studies – referral patterns, failure to enter treatment and attrition. Pain 43: 7–25
Turk D C, Rudy T E 1991 Neglected topics in the treatment of chronic pain patients – relapse, noncompliance, and adherence enhancement. Pain 44: 5–28
Turner J A 1982 Comparison of group progressive relaxation training and cognitive-behavioral group therapy for chronic low back pain. Journal of Consulting and Clinical Psychology 50: 757–765
Ulen S S, Armsborg T J 1992 A strategy for evaluating occupational risk factors of musculoskeletal disorders. Journal of Occupational Rehabilitation 2: 35–50
Woolf C J 1989 Recent advances in the pathophysiology of acute pain. British Journal of Anaesthetics 63: 139–146

SECTION 2

Occupational therapy concerns

Section 2 begins with an examination of occupational therapy practice models for pain management and continues with a brief look at assessment issues. Treatment concerns for the occupational therapist are then discussed.

SECTION CONTENTS

4. Occupational therapy involvement in pain management   43

5. Assessment issues   71

6. Scope of occupational therapy treatment   93

7. Treatment issues – techniques for pain management   117

8. Special treatment topics   139

4

Occupational therapy involvement in pain management

Occupational therapists and pain associations 44
The literature 44
　The role of the occupational therapist 45
　Summary 50
Models of practice 51
　The biopsychosocial model 51
　The occupational behaviour model 52
　The model of human occupation 56

The operant conditioning/ behavioural model 60
The attitude–beliefs–intentions– behaviour model 61
The appraisal model of coping 63
The commonsense model of illness 64
My preferred model 65
Chapter summary 67
References 68

The occupational therapist works within the multidisciplinary framework to rehabilitate patients to an improved quality of life and to assist patients in attaining and maintaining a sense of task mastery and competence (Strong 1984).

Given the magnitude of the difficulties faced by many individuals with pain, and particularly the disruption which pain effects within the individual's life, it would seem clear to me, as an occupational therapist, that it is essential for pain management teams to include an occupational therapist as one of the core health professionals. However, such a need has not been seen so clearly by others. As recently as 1990, Nanci I Moore wrote: 'Few descriptions of pain teams include the role of the occupational therapist' (Moore 1990). A cursory examination of many of the basic pain books reveals that many frequently fail to mention occupational therapy as part of the treatment armamentum for pain patients (see, for example, Burrows et al 1987 and Camic & Brown 1989). Other books, such as the definitive *Textbook of Pain*, by Wall and Melzack (1994) make mention of occupational therapy, but have no specific chapter devoted to it (in contrast, three chapters in the *Textbook of Pain* concern physiotherapy).

In this chapter therefore, an investigation will be made into the extent of current occupational therapy involvement in pain management. We begin by examining membership categories of the multidisciplinary pain associations of the International Association of the Study of Pain (IASP), the Australian Pain Society (APS), the New Zealand Pain Society (NZPS), the Canadian Pain Society, the American Pain Society and the British and Irish Pain Society, to determine the number of occupational therapy members. Then, an examination is made of the occupational therapy literature, so that the reader can become acquainted with the depth and volume of literature on and by occupational therapists on the topic of pain management. Occupational therapy practice models for pain management are then considered and illustrated using case examples. The model which guides my own practice in pain management is then described. The unique and valued contribution which the occupational therapist can make to helping people with chronic pain is thus examined in this chapter.

OCCUPATIONAL THERAPISTS AND PAIN ASSOCIATIONS

Pain associations are organizations established to help improve the management of patients with pain problems and to foster research into pain. Hence, it may be beneficial for occupational therapists to belong to such organizations. Foremost amongst such organizations is the International Association for the Study of Pain (IASP). IASP members include basic scientists, physicians and health professionals from a variety of disciplines (IASP 1993). The 1993 Membership Directory of IASP identifies 12 occupational therapy members, drawn from Australia, Canada, Colombia, New Zealand, Sweden, and the USA. The Australian Pain Society has 13 members who are occupational therapists, out of a total membership of 527 (2.5% of membership are occupational therapists), while the New Zealand Pain Society has 16 occupational therapists amongst its 210 members (7.6%).

Certainly these figures suggest that occupational therapists form only a small part of all pain societies. However, there is usually some representation. It is interesting to note that the International Association for the Study of Pain has acknowledged the contribution of occupational therapy to pain management with its 1995 publication of the undergraduate pain curriculum for occupational therapists and physiotherapists (Unruh et al 1994).

THE LITERATURE

A literature search was undertaken in a number of ways. First, all occupational therapy literature gathered in an ad hoc way over a 15-year period was examined. This ad hoc procedure tapped both refereed journals and non-refereed conference proceedings. A total of 61 papers were retrieved in this way. Secondly, a systematic search of the literature of the past 10 years was made by means of MedLine and PsychLit computer retrieval searches, using the keywords of occupational therapy and pain. An additional three papers were retrieved in this way.

Topics covered in the literature have shown a developmental progression, moving from the delineation of the occupational therapy role (Caruso & Chan 1986, Flower et al 1981, Strong 1987), to documentation of practice extent (Strong 1986a, Wyrick et al 1991), and treatment efficacy studies (Tyson & Strong 1990).

In this chapter, we examine the literature on the delineation of role chronologically and in detail; the literature pertaining to practice issues and research on treatment effectiveness will be considered in subsequent chapters on occupational therapy treatment (Chs 6, 7, 8).

The role of the occupational therapist

Grant (1978) commented 'The inception of Occupational Therapy within the Pain Relief Clinic followed a few isolated encounters with pain relief cases on the ward. The continued expansion has been a response to a growing awareness of patient needs which can be met by Occupational Therapy services'. Her Australian conference paper was the first written description I have found of occupational therapy services within a pain relief clinic. Patients typically seen in this setting had conditions such as back and neck pain, cancer pain, phantom limb pain, causalgia, neuropathic pain, sympathetic dystrophy or post-trauma pain. Occupational therapy for these patients included early mobilization after procedures such as nerve blocks, functional assessments, work simplification, work assessment, assessment for electrode implants, recreational and avocational activities, discussion groups, relaxation and spouses' groups.

Chronic spinal pain

The next description of occupational therapy and pain management was from the United States of America (Flower et al 1981). A multidisciplinary approach to treating patients with chronic spinal pain was described; the role of the occupational therapist in such a program is illustrated in Figure 4.1. It can be seen that the skills of both the physical occupational therapist and the psychosocial occupational therapist were utilized by such a program. Goals of occupational therapy assessment in the first treatment phase were to evaluate home and vocational activities of the patient, and to observe physical and emotional responses to stressful activities, activity tolerances, body mechanics and pain reporting. Treatment goals in this phase were to educate the patient about the spine, body mechanics, posture and relaxation. The second phase of treatment was directed towards increasing the patient's physical activity, defining problems and goal setting for discharge.

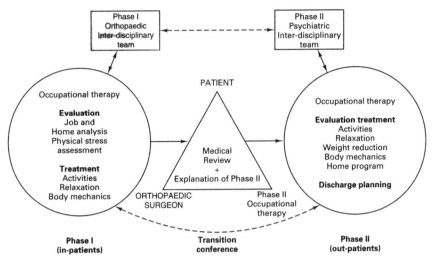

Figure 4.1 The role of occupational therapy in a chronic spinal pain program. (Adapted from Flower et al 1981, with permission. © AOTA)

Aims for occupational therapy intervention

At the 1984 Australian Association of Occupational Therapists Federal Conference, two occupational therapists outlined the role of the occupational therapist with patients with pain. Mangiamele (1984) identified eight aims for occupational therapy intervention, as follows:

1. Evaluating how the pain affects the patient's life.
2. Helping the patient to gain greater self-understanding.
3. Motivating the patient to be an active player in management.
4. Reducing pain behaviours.
5. Assessing and increasing function.
6. Teaching relaxation and stress management.
7. Developing well behaviours.
8. Setting goals.

Meanwhile, Strong (1984) also identified eight components of the occupational therapy role in pain management. These were:

1. Use of techniques to increase the patient's resumption in valued life activities.
2. Education in correct body mechanics.
3. Training in relaxation techniques.
4. Engagement in groups.
5. Counselling and support.
6. Organization of community-based supports.
7. Staff education.
8. Research.

Johnson (1984) described occupational therapy as providing 'an environmental laboratory' where patients with chronic pain can learn to re-establish competence and control in their lives. The specific contribution which can be made by occupational therapists in pain management is related to role behaviours. The occupational therapist can assist the patient to understand the impact of pain on her daily life, can help to re-establish a daily schedule, and can help to increase physical activity (Johnson 1984). The use of goal-directed groups was also considered important.

Blakeney (1984) described the occupational therapist's work with patients with chronic pain presenting to a pain clinic in the United States of America. The aim of such intervention was to examine the patient's occupational performance, and to help her to establish a balance of activity as it relates to work, self-care and play. Meanwhile, Tigges et al (1984) identified the goal of occupational therapy with patients in a hospice setting as reducing 'the pain of loss of role'.

Extent of occupational therapy involvement

In 1986, the results of a survey of the extent of occupational therapy involvement in pain management in Queensland, Australia, were published (Strong 1986a). A questionnaire posted to all 385 occupational therapists registered in the state of Queensland in 1985 yielded a 50% response rate. A third of respondents worked, to a greater or lesser extent, with patients with chronic pain. Yet all of these therapists also held responsibility for another caseload. In fact, 78% of therapists reported spending less than 5 hours per week treating pain patients. Only 14% of the occupational therapists worked as part of a multidisciplinary pain clinic, with the other 86% of respondents seeing patients with pain as part of a general caseload or in a unit such as a rheumatology clinic. Patients seen included those with back pain, arthritis, headache, cancer, abdominal pain, thalamic pain, phantom limb pain, post-herpetic neuralgia and psychogenic pain. Occupational therapists reported using treatment strategies such as activities of daily living, prescription of assistive devices, work simplification, counselling, relaxation, body mechanics, splinting, stress management, avocational training, group activities and work assessment (Strong 1986a).

US chronic pain management program

Giles and Allen (1986) discussed the occupational therapy role in treating patients admitted to a chronic pain management program in the United States of America. Types of patients seen included those with low back pain, headache, cervical pain, causalgia, arthritis, cancer, internal pain and pain with no identifiable lesion. The goal of this program was to help patients realize that they have some control over pain, and to help patients to improve their quality of life. Treatment strategies implemented included education in energy conservation, work simplification, body mechanics, joint protection, relaxation, biofeedback, use of transcutaneous nerve stimulation, prescription of adaptive equipment, work assessment, recreation and strengthening activity programs.

US acute back pain therapy program

Meanwhile, an occupational therapy program in the United States of America for patients with acute back pain was documented by Caruso and Chan (1986). Key treatment was focused upon similar strategies to those listed above, in programs directed towards patients with chronic pain. The occupational therapy goal for patients with acute back pain was to 'facilitate the development of problem-solving skills through patient education and training' (Caruso & Chan 1986). An early intervention program designed to return employees with work-related back pain to work was then described (Caruso et al 1987). Treatment consisted of education on back protection and its application to the home and work settings, job evaluation, work hardening, exercise and relaxation.

Contribution of occupational therapists to pain management

The first paper to be delivered by an occupational therapist at an Australian Pain Society Annual Scientific Meeting was presented in 1986 (Strong 1986b). Since then, occupational therapists have been regular presenters at these annual scientific meetings, with topics ranging from task performance and occupational overuse injuries (Sikorski & Molan 1987), to patient assessment (Strong & Ashton 1992), and the use of groups in pain management (Pritchard 1991).

The occupational therapy role in chronic pain management was further reinforced by Strong (1987), who described the presence of chronic pain as interfering with the patient's successful performance of activities of daily living. Treatment strategies used by the occupational therapist with such patients were activities of daily living, body mechanics, stress management, activity prescription, counselling and work assessment.

Lloyd and Coggles (1988) reported on the occupational therapy contribution to pain management for women with metastatic breast disease. The occupational therapist was described as assisting individual patients to become as independent as possible in personally relevant life roles.

A further report on the role of the occupational therapist in pain management (Strong 1989) again identified key contributions of the occupational therapist as increasing the patient's functional independence, engendering feelings of self-responsibility in the patient regarding her well-being, increasing self-esteem, and assisting in pain control.

Purposeful activity and pain reduction

A somewhat different role for occupational therapy in pain management was identified by McCormack (1988): 'The occupational therapist can contribute to pain management by providing non-invasive techniques and purposeful activities that have been shown to potentiate physiological mechanisms associated with pain reduction'. By engaging patients in purposeful activity, physiological mechanisms associated with pain reduction can be stimulated. It is suggested that patients first be introduced to enabling activities such as relaxation, cutaneous stimulation and cognitive distraction prior to engagement in purposeful activity. Wynn Parry (1982, 1983) observed a similar function of purposeful activity when he spoke about pain management for patients with brachial plexus avulsion lesions. He suggested that engagement in purposeful activity may help to activate a patient's inhibition of spontaneously firing dorsal horn cells. He said: 'When patients are totally absorbed in work or hobbies the pain can abate or even disappear altogether, thus return to realistic work as soon as possible after brachial plexus lesions is the most effective way of helping these patients' pain' (Wynn Parry 1982). In a similar vein to McCormack, Heck (1990) has identified the strategies of distraction, relaxation and cutaneous stimulation as being of value in decreasing the adverse effects of acute pain upon the patient's activities.

Occupational therapy and HIV infection

Galantino (1990) described a role for both physical and occupational therapists in assisting patients with HIV infection, suggesting that they 'conduct pain assessments and evaluate functional impairment to better employ non-invasive techniques for management of HIV complications'. No distinction was made between the tasks of the physical therapist and the occupational therapist. The areas specified for intervention included manual therapy, neuromuscular re-education, use of modalities, cognitive distraction, exercise intervention, endurance training, nutritional advice and psychological intervention.

Occupational therapy in UK pain clinic

O'Hara (1992), in reporting on her role as a full-time occupational therapist in a British pain clinic, identified many of the tasks and functions previously reported. They encompassed group work, seating prescription, functional assessment, patient education, and research. Patients seen included those with back pain, cancer pain and reflex sympathetic dystrophy. O'Hara commented on the difficulties faced by many sessional and part-time occupational therapists in pain management. Surprisingly, she also commented upon the lack of a specific role for the occupational therapist within the team structure. Given that several papers were written in the 1980s on the occupational therapy role, it is probable that the role difficulty for the occupational therapist may have arisen more from other team members' uncertainty than from professional self-doubt.

Dual practice of occupational therapy

This difficulty in articulating exactly what it is that we (occupational therapists) do with patients has been eloquently discussed by Mattingly and Fleming (1994) in their examination of the clinical reasoning of occupational therapists. They described the dual practice of occupational therapy, and the tendency for occupational therapists to document and discuss the biomedical aspects of their practice, while continuing with what they call their underground practice of helping patients to adjust to and live with their illness. In the pain management literature reviewed thus far, the existence of two levels of practice can be seen. For example, Mangiamele (1984) talked of helping patients to understand how the pain has affected their lives, Strong (1989) discussed helping engender within patients the feeling of self-responsibility, and Johnson (1984) mentioned providing the environment where patients can learn to re-establish competence. At the same time, authors described the use of techniques such as the prescription of adaptive equipment (see, for example, Caruso & Chan 1986), and body mechanics education (see, for example, Strong 1986a). This dual focus of occupational therapy practice will be discussed further later in this chapter.

Summary

The occupational therapy literature spanning three decades has provided a consistent picture of occupational therapists providing services for people with a variety of pain problems. Common themes to emerge are the occupational therapist's concern with maximizing the patient's functional status and control over her life, and minimizing the patient's loss of role and associated competences. Additionally, some occupational therapists are working to control pain, both acute and chronic, through specific techniques and engagement in purposeful activity.

Not all occupational therapists work full-time in pain management programs. Such multiple caseload constraints may limit the type and extent of occupational therapy services in pain management programs. Nevertheless, this reading of the occupational therapy literature reveals a contribution which can be made by the occupational therapist. The value of such a contribution may be better understood by now considering the models which guide the practice of occupational therapists when working with patients with pain.

MODELS OF PRACTICE

Drawing from the American Occupational Therapy Association's Clinical Reasoning Study, Mattingly (1994) observed that the work of occupational therapists frequently has two orientations; one which examines the meaning of the illness upon the person's life, and the other which treats that same patient's body as a separate physical entity. The acknowledgement that illness is a distinctive experience for patients is an important component of occupational therapy (Moss-Morris & Petrie 1994). An examination of both occupational therapy literature and occupational therapy practice in pain management reveals a similar confluence and/or disjuncture between helping patients to adjust to life with pain, and treating patients with a biomechanical approach. There are many things which occupational therapists do to/for patients with pain problems, from giving them cushions to desensitizing painful body areas. Yet, it is rare for such technical treatment to form the sole contribution of the occupational therapist to that patient. Occupational therapy treatment is typically more holistic.

What are the predominant models which guide the practice of occupational therapy in pain management? In this section, the prominent practice models articulated/identified by occupational therapists for pain management work will be explained, and illustrated using case examples. The models to be considered are the biopsychosocial model (Milne 1983), the occupational behaviour model (Blakeney 1984, Strong 1989, Tigges et al 1984), the model of human occupation (Gusich 1984, Kielhofner & Burke 1980), the operant/behavioural model (Engel 1990, Giles & Allen 1986), the attitude–beliefs–intentions–behaviour model (Fishbein & Ajzen 1975), the appraisal model of coping (Gage 1992), and the commonsense model of illness (Moss-Morris & Petrie 1994).

The biopsychosocial model

The biopsychosocial model takes into consideration the body, mind and environment of the individual (Cronin Mosey 1974). Proposed by Engel (1978, 1980) as an extension of the biomedical model, the biopsychosocial model was advocated as a useful model for guiding occupational therapy practice (Cronin Mosey 1974). An important assumption of the model is that the individual has the right to a meaningful and productive life, even in the face of a chronic disease (Cronin Mosey 1974). Cronin Mosey felt that the model was useful for occupational therapists 'because it focuses upon man as a biological entity, a thinking and feeling person, and a member of a community of others'.

Milne (1983), a New Zealand occupational therapist, has described the application of the biopsychosocial model to a multidisciplinary pain management program. The program consisted of interventions which addressed the biological, psychological and social aspects of the patient and her pain. Biological treatment was concerned with educating the patient about her pain, thereby demystifying the pain experience. Ways to modify the pain could then be taught. Psychological treatment considered the influence of psychological factors on the patient's pain. Finally, the effect of the social environment on the patient would then be considered.

Appraisal of the model

The biopsychosocial model is useful in that it widens our view of the patient with pain – we no longer view the pain as a biological symptom which exists in isolation from all other aspects of the person. The impact on, and interaction between the patient's pain and other individuals in the patient's environment can be examined using this model. However, while providing a useful peg on which to hang many facets of the patient's pain, the model fails to explain the type of assessment tools to be used by the therapist, or the specific types of interventions required to effect change. Additionally, the mechanisms by which the relative importance of various factors may be assessed is not made clear. Nevertheless, the biopsychosocial model has clear advantages over the biomedical model, as the case example in Box 4.1 illustrates.

The occupational behaviour model

Order in occupational therapy has been conceptualized as competence in occupational performance (Rogers 1982). As noted by Blakeney (1984), 'occupational behaviour provides a very useful frame of reference for an occupational therapist treating the chronic pain patient'. The occupational behaviour model sees patients as people with particular life roles who experience both assets and difficulties in their performance of the activities of daily living (Matsutsuyu 1971). Occupational therapists believe that human beings require a balance between work, self-care, rest, play and sleep (Matsutsuyu 1971). For patients with pain, the pain may interfere with any one aspect, or with several aspects of occupation. Of particular importance then, to an occupational therapist, is an assessment of the

> **Box 4.1** The case of Mrs D
>
> Mrs D was a 50-year-old woman who presented to pain clinic, suffering from severe anterior chest wall pain subsequent to bilateral mastectomies. In occupational therapy, her occupational therapist was not so much concerned with the biological aspect of her pain and its management; the biological management was being undertaken by other team members. The occupational therapist focused more on the psychological and social aspects of Mrs D's problem. Mrs D had been fitted with tear-drop prostheses after her mastectomies, but she was not using them when seen in occupational therapy. It transpired that there were two problems in wearing the prostheses: first, it hurt Mrs D to do up her bra, and second, even if she did manage to get the bra done up, the prostheses never stayed in place, causing her embarrassment and anxiety. So, the prime intervention in occupational therapy was to remedy this situation. Velcro was sewn to her prostheses and to the inside of the bra cups. The hook and eye fastening was also changed to a velcro fastening. Mrs D could now put the prostheses in place before putting on the bra, and she could now manage to do up the velcro closure without too much pain. Mrs D was happy with these modifications, which did not greatly alter her pain, but which greatly enhanced her self-image and self-confidence. This, in turn, facilitated her greater participation in daily life.

activity levels, activity patterns and functional status of patients with pain. The areas of self-care, work, rest and play are each considered (Blakeney 1984, Strong 1989). 'Many chronic pain patients relinquish various daily living tasks because of pain, with a resultant occupational dysfunction' (Strong 1989). The relinquishment of these tasks or occupations by the patient can lead to considerable imbalance in that person's life, and can compound the initial pain problem. It is not hard to understand how the patient with pain can get caught in a maladaptive pain cycle, with non-performance in particular domains undermining self-confidence, personal autonomy and life roles. Such negative consequences are often concomitant with decreased physical condition and decreased activity tolerance, making performance even more difficult. Figure 4.2 illustrates such a pain cycle.

The patient in such a cycle may feel that her difficulties are insurmountable. When patients with pain problems are seen by occupational therapists, they are often already well into the pain cycle. As such, they typically present with role loss or, at the very least, some level of role interference, decreased physical activity and decreased self-esteem.

Intervention by the occupational therapist begins with a thorough assessment of the client's current and past occupational history and performance. This assessment will include a work history, a play/leisure history, a self-care evaluation, an examination of daily activity levels, and an assessment of avocational and vocational skills and interests (Blakeney 1984). As well as the past history and current status of the client, an appreciation of their patient's future goals is also important (Blakeney 1984).

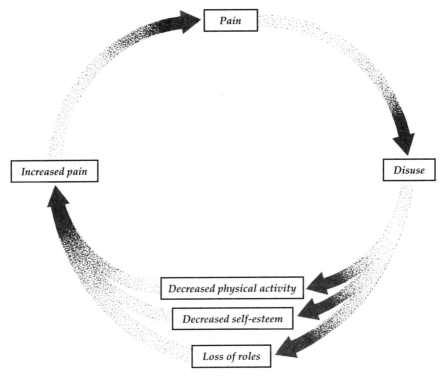

Figure 4.2 Chronic pain cycle. (© Adis International 1996. First published in Patient Management Australia, September 1989. Reproduced with permission.)

Intervention by the occupational therapist can help to break the chronic pain cycle (see Fig. 4.3). Despite the continuation of the pain, the patient is able to regain some of the balance lost between the personally relevant occupational activities in her life, which, in turn, can lead to an improvement in quality of life for the patient.

Appraisal of the model

The occupational behaviour model provides a holistic picture of the patient with chronic pain, as well as some tools for a more comprehensive assessment of patients with pain. Such instruments as the NPI interest checklist (Matsutsuyu 1969), or the modified interest checklist (Rogers 1988), and the occupational history (Moorehead 1969) can elicit useful information. Further, the model provides a focus for occupational therapy intervention, with its emphasis on re-establishing order in the occupational functioning of the individual patient.

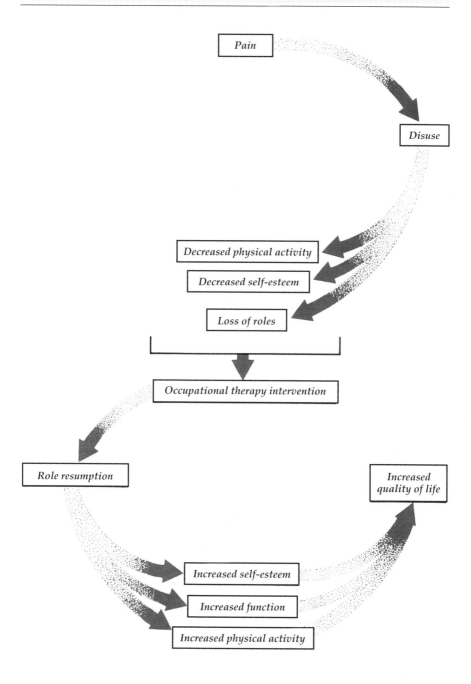

Figure 4.3 Occupational therapy interruption to the chronic pain cycle. (© Adis International 1996. First published in Patient Management Australia, September 1989. Reproduced with permission.)

> **Box 4.2** The case of Ms J
>
> Ms J was referred to the occupational therapist by the anaesthetics consultant. When seen by the occupational therapist, Ms J was an in-patient at the local hospital. Ms J was a 25-year-old woman, who, 5 years previously, had contracted Guillain–Barré syndrome, during which time she had required treatment in an intensive care unit. After a period of rehabilitation, Ms J had returned to her job. On presentation to the occupational therapist, her pain consisted of dysasthesic pain in both lower limbs, which made wearing shoes unbearable, and prolonged walking and standing difficult. She also had lumbar and cervical back pain.
>
> Ms J's occupational history showed a high level of performance. She had completed high school and commenced work in a government job (defence force). On recovering from Guillain–Barré syndrome, she had returned to this employment. Prior to her hospitalization, she had been working, but with increasing difficulty. Her job required a high level of physical fitness, with daily physical activities. She needed to stand for long periods, and to wear regulation footwear. Another task which she described as difficult involved a great deal of bending. An additional problem she was experiencing at work was the difficulty her colleagues had in understanding her limitations. They had been prepared to make allowances for someone who had just been seriously ill with Guillain–Barré syndrome, but had difficulty in understanding that she could not carry out all her tasks with ease, even though her muscles had recovered. Ms J reported her desire to continue working in her current job.
>
> Social history indicated that Ms J was in a steady relationship and was contemplating having a child, but was concerned that she would not be able to cope with motherhood, given the limitations placed upon her by pain. She currently was not able to perform many domestic tasks; her usual pattern was to arrive home from work and collapse in a heap.
>
> Occupational therapy treatment with Ms J was directed towards a number of goals. First, a desensitization program was trialled to increase her ability to wear shoes and to stand on her feet. Alternative types of footwear were explored. Second, Ms J was educated about work simplification techniques and good body mechanics as they applied to activities of daily living, domestic activities, motherhood activities, and work activities. Third, a worksite visit was conducted, and Ms J's jobs, routines and environment were assessed. Modifications to tasks, routines and environment were recommended to enhance Ms J's ability to function to her maximum capability.

A case example showing how an occupational therapist was guided by the occupational behaviour model is given in Box 4.2.

The model of human occupation

Like the occupational behaviour model, the model of human occupation is based on the assumption that occupation is crucial for the individual (Kielhofner & Burke 1980). The individual is seen as an open system interacting with the environment through human occupation. Three subsystems are seen as integral to the individual, these being volition, habituation and performance. Volition relates to the individual's motivation to engage or do, and comprises the individual's personal causation, valued goals and interests (Kielhofner & Burke 1980). Habituation refers to the patterns or routines which determine occupational behaviour. Of particular note here are the individual's habits and roles (Kielhofner & Burke 1980). Performance relates to the individual's ability to produce skilled actions. The model is illustrated diagrammatically in Figure 4.4.

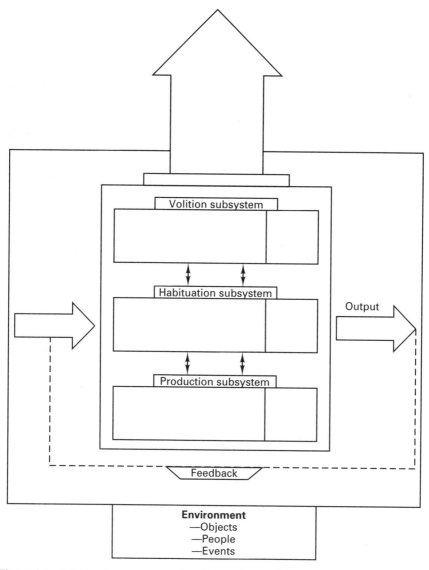

Figure 4.4 A model of human occupation. (Adapted from Kielhofner & Burke 1980, with permission. © AOTA)

Kielhofner (1980), and Smith (1974) before him, have discussed cycles of interaction which occur between the individual (the system) and the environment. Either benign or vicious cycles can occur – a cycle which supports adaptation is called a benign cycle, while a cycle which challenges adaptation is called a vicious cycle. A patient's participation in either of these cycles will be dependent upon her internal beliefs along with her experiences of success or failure (Kielhofner 1980).

Model of human occupation and the chronic pain cycle

Gusich (1984) identified a chronic pain cycle in which patients with chronic pain could become entrapped. Guided by the model of human occupation, the therapist considers the individual patient's functioning in terms of the three subsystems. As Smith (1974) so eloquently stated, 'The therapeutic task is to transform the vicious spiral of helplessness and hopelessness into a benign one, enhancing the patient's agency'.

Using the model of human occupation, the goal of the occupational therapist is still to enhance the patient's occupational behaviour (Gusich 1984). Evaluation of each patient takes into consideration the patient's status in the three subsystems of volition, habituation and performance, as well as the environment, and the stages of output, throughput and feedback (Kielhofner et al 1980). Assessments undertaken may include use of measures such as the NPI checklist (Matsutsuyu 1969), the role checklist (Barris et al 1988), and the occupational history (Moorehead 1969). Cubie and Kaplan (1982) have provided a series of questions based upon the model of human occupation which can be useful in evaluating the individual's occupational behaviour. These questions are:

- Does the client perform work, play and self-care behaviours competently and consistently?
- What does the client value?
- What are the client's interests?
- Does the client anticipate success in the performance of daily life tasks?
- Can the client identify productive occupational roles?
- Does the client have organized habit patterns?
- Does the client have the necessary skills to carry out work, play, and self-care activities?
- Does the physical environment support competent and consistent use of skills?
- Does the social environment require occupational roles that the client enjoys and performs well?
- Does the social environment support successful occupational behaviour?

Appraisal of the model

The model of human occupation is a useful one to guide the practice of occupational therapists in pain management. It provides an understanding of order and disorder in the individual, many of the tools to assess function, and a framework for assisting individual patients to maximize their occupational performance. The case example in Box 4.3 illustrates how an occupational therapist working with the model of human occupation can help patients with chronic pain.

Box 4.3 The case of Mrs P (First published in Patient Management Australia, September 1989. © Adis International 1995. Presented with permission.)

Mrs P was a 50-year-old woman who had suffered from chronic intractable pain for the past 12 years. Her 65-year-old husband had retired from his job 5 years previously to care for her. Prior to her admission to hospital, Mrs P had been confined to bed, getting up only to toilet, shower, and visit the doctor. Mrs P's pain was facial pain, due to post-herpetic neuralgia in the distribution of her trigeminal nerve.

A summary of her occupational therapy assessment shows that Mrs P had:

1. lost feelings of personal causation; she had low self-esteem and poor self-confidence
2. lost her interests of tennis, gardening, craft, reading, and domestic activities
3. lost her valued goal of being a good wife
4. relinquished her primary and secondary roles of homemaker and spouse; her husband performed all domestic, shopping and gardening activities, and cared for her
5. adopted the invalid role
6. no physical limitations; she was physically mobile, but was deconditioned and had decreased activity tolerance due to disuse
7. good performance skills, but she was not using them; she had been employed as a waitress and cook prior to her marriage, and had been a competent homemaker prior to the onset of the shingles
8. no demands being made upon her; the social environment was contributing to her illness behaviour.

The occupational therapy treatment program was based on the following aims for Mrs P:

1. to increase her self-esteem and self-confidence
2. to re-activate her interests
3. to re-establish her occupational roles of homemaker and spouse
4. to eliminate her invalid role
5. to re-establish her use of performance skills
6. to reduce her social isolation.

Mrs P had a 2-week stay in the pain management unit, during which time she was seen daily by the occupational therapist and the physiotherapist. The initial treatment modality chosen by the occupational therapist was Mrs P's previously good performance skills as a cook. Using the pretext that the therapist was unable to cook, Mrs P was asked to help to bake a cake for someone on her ward. She needed much reassurance during the session, but was very pleased when she successfully produced a cake which was admired by and devoured by all in the ward. She quickly

> **Box 4.3 cont'd**
>
> progressed to preparing her own lunch and that of another patient she had befriended. As her confidence in her cooking skills and her ability to have some positive effect upon her environment grew, she gained the confidence to try engaging in other activities, both on the ward and in occupational therapy. As a bonus, as her activity level grew and her feelings of competence increased, her ability to manage her pain increased.
>
> On discharge, Mrs P still had pain, for which she now used a TENS unit provided by the physiotherapist, but she was no longer invalided by it. She had been enabled to become an active participant in life. Discharge follow-up was arranged with the local general practitioner and the local hospital therapist. It was felt that Mrs P and her husband might need ongoing support, both to reinforce her new well behaviour, and to help him to adjust to the changes he would need to experience in his life.

The operant conditioning/behavioural model

A number of authors have suggested that occupational therapists might include aspects of the operant conditioning model in their practice in pain management (see for example, Blakeney 1984, Engel 1990, Giles & Allen 1986). Since this model was covered in some detail in Chapter 3, only those components which relate directly to occupational therapy practice will be considered here. One of the central tenets of this model is that pain behaviours of patients with chronic pain may be perpetuated by environmental reinforcers such as attention or avoidance of disliked activities (Giles & Allen 1986). Giles and Allen (1986) have suggested that occupational therapists can use operant principles by 'making attention and approval contingent upon "well behaviours" '.

Appraisal of the model

Blakeney (1984) has suggested that the occupational therapy focus on occupational role performance of the patient is compatible with a behavioural approach. However, one does not need to search too far to find areas where occupational therapy management of patients with chronic pain and operant principles reach an impasse (Strong 1990). For example, Engel (1990) raised as an issue the conflict between prescribing adaptive equipment for patients with chronic pain (see Tyson & Strong 1990), and the principles of operant pain management programs. As Engel quite rightly identifies, one of the goals of operant programs is to reduce and eliminate external approaches (or 'crutches') to pain control, such as medication use, or walking stick use, or cushion use. This certainly sets up a conflict with a large portion of occupational therapy practice!

The detailed focus by occupational therapists on the meaning of pain in a person's life is also a practice not promoted by an operant approach. An

> **Box 4.4** An operant approach
>
> Cardenas et al (1986) reported on the use of a behavioural program with a 37-year-old woman with chronic pain and hysterical right arm paralysis. In occupational therapy, the patient was helped to set goals for the use of her arm, and baseline data on her arm and hand function were obtained. The patient then began a daily hand-exercise program, which contained a number of step-wise increments. As each increment or quota was attained, the patient was praised. It was reported that after 1 month, the patient had attained normal hand function scores, and therapy ceased.

extension of this, and another area of possible discord between the occupational therapy approach and the operant approach, is the detailed initial assessment made by the occupational therapist. The therapist will try to determine what the pain is like and how and to what degree the pain limits the patient's activities. I have frequently been challenged by occupational therapists at conferences when I have called for a detailed and comprehensive assessment to be made of the patient and their pain. 'Is not that contrary to an operant approach?' I have been asked. My reply has been that to work effectively with patients with chronic pain, I must first have a full understanding of their pain and its effect upon the many facets of their life. To deny patients' pain, and to look only at increasing their activity levels seems to me to be less than holistic.

Given these provisos, there are a number of goals of the operant approach which do fit nicely with an occupational therapy approach, these being to reduce pain behaviours, to increase activity levels, and to restore well behaviours (Turk & Rudy 1988). Vlaeyen and his colleagues (1989) described an operant program which was conducted within occupational therapy and physiotherapy, with psychology support, for a woman with chronic low back pain. This program aimed to increase the patient's sitting and standing tolerances.

The case example in Box 4.4 illustrates the treatment of a patient with chronic pain using an operant approach. Since I do not operate from a strictly behavioural framework, the case example is drawn from the work of an occupational therapist (Larson) and colleagues (Cardenas et al 1986).

The attitude–beliefs–intentions–behaviour model

In recent years, attitude–behaviour relations have been increasingly examined in the pain management literature (Jensen & Karoly 1987, Jensen et al 1987, Riley et al 1988, Schwartz et al 1985, Shutty et al 1990, Strong et al 1992, Williams & Thorn 1989) and in the occupational therapy literature (Gage 1992, Moss-Morris & Petrie 1994, Strong et al 1990). Many authors have called for the routine evaluation of a pain patient's attitudes towards and beliefs about her pain and its management (Strong et al 1992, Williams & Thorn 1989). Turk and Rudy (1992) commented: 'Patients' beliefs, appraisals, and expectations about their pain, their ability to cope, their social supports, their disorder, the medicolegal system, the healthcare system, and their employers are all important as they may facilitate or disrupt the patient's sense of control and ability to manage pain'.

Attitudes are the predispositions people have to respond in a consistent way to an object, which in this case is pain (Ajzen 1988, Fishbein & Ajzen 1975). Beliefs are the information which an individual knows about the object (Fishbein & Ajzen 1975). Pain beliefs, then, represent the person's individual understanding of what the pain is and what it means to them (Williams & Thorn 1989).

Fishbein and Ajzen's model

Fishbein and Ajzen (1975) have provided a model of the relationship between beliefs, attitudes, intentions and behaviours towards an object, which can be useful when considering a person with pain. The model posits that beliefs are the information an individual has about their pain, while attitudes are learned predispositions to act in a certain way regarding their pain. From a person's attitudes will arise intentions towards performing particular behaviours (see, for example, the case of Mrs V in Box 4.5). (This particular model has not identified specific assessment tools to be used in evaluating attitudes and beliefs. In Chapter 5, measures suitable for evaluating attitudes and beliefs will be discussed.)

Box 4.5 The case of Mrs V

Mrs V was a 45-year-old woman with chronic low back pain of 3 years' duration. She believed that if she bent her back, then her L5–S1 fusion would 'snap'. Her attitude towards doing any bending was very negative. It was her intention not to do any activity which required her to bend. Hence, her resultant behaviour was that she did not do any housework which involved bending.

Since this model does allow for the possibility of feedback and learning, there are a number of ways therapists can use it to facilitate change. Consider the first part of the model, the beliefs section, as it relates to the patient Mrs V. Remember that beliefs are the information that a person has about her pain, and in Mrs V's case, her fusion. If Mrs V was given more information about what the 'fusion' is, how it was performed, and what it means in terms of the joint integrity, then Mrs V's beliefs about her fusion and activity might change. This might, in turn, modify her attitudes, intentions and subsequent behaviour.

Consider also the behaviour part of the model. If, with the support and supervision of the occupational therapist, Mrs V was able to complete some domestic activities which required her to bend her back, and her fusion did not break, then her beliefs might also be modified by this behaviour.

> **Box 4.6** The case of Mr G
>
> Mr G was a 44-year-old man who was admitted to pain clinic with chronic low back pain. He had been in pain for 7 years, subsequent to sustaining a lifting injury at work. He had been invalided out of the workforce, and was now on an invalid pension. Radiological examinations had found no observable abnormality. He had not had any surgery for his low back pain.
>
> Mr G presented as a man displaying minimal distress. He had a low pain intensity, a low depression score, and a low percentage of body area in pain. However, he reported that the pain was interfering greatly in the performance of his activities of daily living, particularly instrumental activities. When assessed on the Survey of Pain Attitudes Revised scale (Jensen et al 1987), Mr G had elevated scores on the Medical Cure scale, the Disability scale and the Desires Solicitude scale, and lower scores on the Emotional Link scale. It could be said that his attitudes were dysfunctional for a chronic pain rehabilitation program. Mr G seemed much more interested in an acute pain management model. Indeed, Mr G later underwent surgery at another facility, despite the absence of clear indicators for surgery during this admission.

The case example in Box 4.6 further illustrates how the attitudes–behaviour framework can guide understanding and practice in pain management.

The appraisal model of coping

Gage (1992) has provided a model to 'guide occupational therapy intervention with respect to assisting patients to cope better with the effects of their disease'. The model is illustrated in Figure 4.5.

Gage's model draws on the work of Lazarus and Folkman (1984) and Bandura (1977, 1982) on coping and self-efficacy respectively. It links an

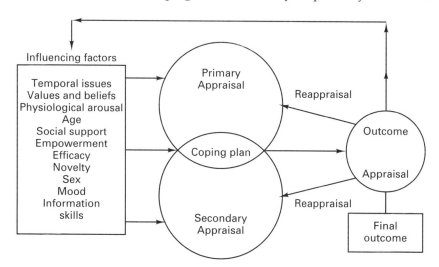

Figure 4.5 The appraisal model of coping. (Adapted from Gage 1992, with permission. © AOTA)

individual's outcomes (such as coping with a disability) with influencing factors (such as beliefs), primary and secondary appraisals, and outcome appraisals. Thus, the interaction between individuals, their environment and their performance is considered. Self-efficacy expectations are the beliefs that individuals have about whether they can successfully perform a particular behaviour required to produce a particular outcome (Bandura 1977, 1982). An outcome expectation is the belief about whether a particular behaviour will result in a certain outcome (Bandura 1977). A person's self-efficacy beliefs can influence behaviour in several ways; for example, whether a person avoids or participates in an activity, and the amount of effort that is made to try an activity (Bandura 1982).

These concepts, which are included in Gage's model, are highly relevant to the area of pain management. For many pain patients, there can be a discrepancy between the level of inactivity and documented physical limitations (Dolce et al 1986). It has been suggested that self-efficacy beliefs may explain the variability between a patient's skill level and her performance outside the clinic (Gage & Polatajko 1994). For example, Dolce (1987) has considered the relationship between self-efficacy and beliefs held by patients with pain about disability. Meanwhile, in their review of the literature pertaining to coping and pain, Jensen and his colleagues (1991) suggested the need for further work in the area of appraisals, coping and adjustment to pain.

Appraisal of the model

Gage has recommended that further attention be given to this model. The application of the model to an individual with pain may prove very useful since it takes into consideration a patient's attitudes, past experiences and cognitive factors such as appraisals, in addition to the actual event, and present performances. It considers the effect of feedback, and the interaction between the patient and her environment. Gage and her colleagues (1994) have developed the Self-Efficacy Gauge to be used as part of this model.

The commonsense model of illness

Moss-Morris and Petrie (1994) have recently suggested that Leventhal's commonsense model of illness (Leventhal et al 1992, Meyer et al 1985) may be a useful adjunct to help occupational therapists understand the meaning of illness in a patient's life. The model is depicted in Figure 4.6.

The commonsense model assumes that the individual is an active processor of illness information, and that such processing involves developing illness representations or beliefs, developing a coping plan, and

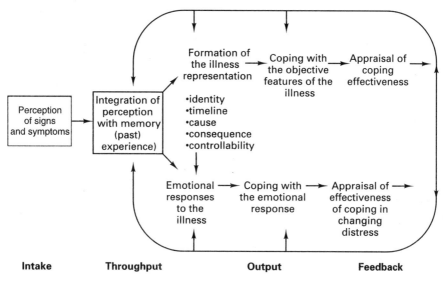

Figure 4.6 The processing stages in the commonsense model of illness in association with the model of human occupation. (Adapted from Moss-Morris & Petrie 1994, with permission.)

appraising coping effectiveness (Moss-Morris & Petrie 1994). In outlining the usefulness of the model to occupational therapists, Moss-Morris and Petrie (1994) cited our pain study (Strong et al 1990) and suggested that illness representations may result in ineffective coping strategies.

My preferred model

My practice of occupational therapy with patients with pain is eclectic. I draw on a number of the models thus far presented, especially the model of human occupation and the attitude–beliefs–intentions–behaviour framework. As the case examples utilizing the biopsychosocial model, the occupational behaviour model, the model of human occupation and the attitude–beliefs–intentions–behaviour model have shown, they all provide useful guidance in understanding and assisting the patient with pain.

In my work I have found the ten guiding questions (p. 58) from the model of human occupation (Cubie & Kaplan 1982) to be helpful in considering the patient's volition, habituation and performance. In terms of the cognitive variables important in adjusting to pain, I am guided by the work on attitudes and behaviour (Fishbein & Ajzen 1975) and coping and appraisals (Lazarus & Folkman 1984). My overall goal in occupational therapy intervention is to assist the person with pain to adjust to living with the chronic condition of pain, and to attain and maintain an optimal level of functioning. Let me share a case example with you (see Box 4.7) which demonstrates my practice.

> **Box 4.7** The case of Mr D
>
> Mr D was a 34-year-old man who presented to pain clinic with a 4-year history of chronic low back pain, bilateral leg pain and generalized body pain. His pain had commenced after a fall at his workplace, where he was employed as a factory hand. Investigations by orthopaedic surgeons had failed to find an operative lesion. After initially receiving workers' compensation benefits, his claim had been settled, and he was now on an invalid pension. On admission, he complained of unbearable pain. Prior to admission, he had been receiving frequent pethidine injections from various doctors in his local community, in addition to taking Panadeine Forte and a large daily intake of muscle relaxant medication. He presented to hospital leaning heavily on a walking stick, and wearing a soft neck-collar. He also had lycra working splints for his hands, and frequently wore the splints during the day.
>
> At the time of his admission to hospital, Mr D described himself as being severely incapacitated in his ability to perform all but the most basic self-care tasks. He described himself as no longer being able to work, perform instrumental daily living activities such as home management, or enjoy himself in any way. He felt that the pain had ruined his life, and until the pain was taken away, his life would not get any better. His partner of 5 years had left him 8 months earlier, and he had moved home to stay with his parents. At home, his mother in particular was responsible for all the cooking, cleaning and shopping, so few demands to perform domestic tasks were placed upon him. His role within the family home was one of a sick visitor. Much of his time was spent idly, with little definite structure in his life.
>
> He identified a number of interests in his life, although he had not pursued any of them much since his injury. He enjoyed playing the guitar, and had been a keen gardener. He had hoped to settle down and have a family, but now he seemed to have no goals, apart from getting rid of his pain.
>
> Mr D presented as a patient with many of the characteristics frequently seen at the pain clinic. He had a multiplicity of problems in his life. These included the physical limitations placed upon him by his pain and the deconditioning process he had undergone over the past 4 years, the enormous losses he had sustained (loss of roles, loss of income security, loss of relationship, loss of valued goal of having a family, and loss of independence), and his belief that while he had pain he was incapacitated.
>
> Using the various models discussed in this chapter, I could have adopted the following approaches:
>
> - From a *biopsychosocial* perspective, I could have embarked upon an education program with Mr D which explained the pain experience. We could then have looked at the effects of his social situation upon his pain, and the influence of psychological factors.
> - Using the *occupational behaviour model*, my focus would have been upon the effects of Mr D's pain on his performance in the domains of work, self-care, rest and play. The role losses incurred could be discussed, as well as planning for future goals. Assistance would then have been given to helping Mr D achieve his occupational goals.
> - An approach guided by the *model of human occupation* would have seen me consider Mr D's volitional, habituation and performance subsystems. Clearly, Mr D has been experiencing problems with all three areas of his life. I would then have worked to help him to improve his occupational behaviour.
> - From an *operant behavioural* point of view, I could have focused upon his many pain behaviours, the overt pain crutches he had adopted and his deconditioning. I could have set him daily activity quotas and thrown away his handsplints.
> - Guided by the *attitude–beliefs–intentions–behaviour model*, I would have carefully examined with Mr D his belief that he was incapacitated as long as he had pain. I would also have carefully examined his other attitudes towards and beliefs about pain. In my therapy, I would then have provided the opportunities for Mr D to realize that he could still achieve certain goals despite pain, along with comprehensive education about pain and the chronic pain cycle.

> **Box 4.7** cont'd
>
> - Using the *appraisal model of coping*, I would have been interested in further exploring Mr D's appraisals about his pain, and his coping strategies to deal with the pain. This would then have formed the basis for a therapy program where I could have provided the opportunities for Mr D to gain a greater sense of self-efficacy by providing him with opportunities for performance accomplishments, exposure to others, adapting to living with pain, and education.
> - Had I been guided by the *commonsense model of illness*, I would have looked further at Mr D's beliefs about his pain, and his current coping strategies.
>
> As it was, I adopted an eclectic approach with Mr D, whereby I did a number of these things. I did look carefully at his performance of work, self-care, play and rest tasks. I did look at his volitional, habituation and performance subsystems, and his future goals. I did plan to reduce his reliance on pain behaviours and to increase his performance of well behaviours. I did carefully examine Mr D's attitudes towards and beliefs about his pain, and look at his appraisals and coping strategies. I also ensured opportunities in my therapy for Mr D to succeed with new adaptive behaviours, thereby increasing his self-efficacy. To have relied on one model alone with Mr D would not, I suggest, have resulted in the most comprehensive and beneficial management program for him.

CHAPTER SUMMARY

In this chapter, I have examined the extent of occupational therapy involvement in, and role in, working with patients with chronic pain. The burgeoning literature is testament to the increasingly evident role for occupational therapists in the pain management area. Given that the primary management goal for patients with chronic pain of non-cancer origin is to rehabilitate them to an improved quality of life independent of the reduction in pain, the contribution of the occupational therapist can be invaluable. Similarly, in the pursuit of the goal of pain reduction and maximizing occupational performance for patients with cancer pain, occupational therapists have much to offer. In their work, occupational therapists can be guided by a number of practice models. This chapter has reviewed the biopsychosocial model, the occupational behaviour model, the model of human occupation, the operant behavioural model, the attitudes–beliefs–intentions–behaviour model, the appraisal model of coping and the commonsense model of illness. Our attention can now be turned to how we should evaluate the patient with pain, and this topic will be the focus of the next chapter.

REFERENCES

Ajzen I 1988 Attitudes, personality, and behaviour. Dorsey Press, Chicago
Bandura A 1977 Self-efficacy: towards a unifying theory of behavioral change. Psychological Review 84: 191–215
Bandura A 1982 Self-efficacy mechanisms in human agency. American Psychologist 37: 122–147
Barris R, Oakley F, Kielhofner G 1988 The role checklist. In: Hemphill B J (ed) Mental health assessment in occupational therapy: an integrative approach to the evaluation process. Slack, Thoroughfare
Blakeney A B 1984 Occupational therapy intervention in chronic pain. Occupational Therapy in Health Care 1: 43–54
Burrows G D, Elton D, Stanley G V 1987 (eds) Handbook of chronic pain management. Elsevier, Amsterdam
Camic P M, Brown F D (eds) 1989 Assessing chronic pain: a multidisciplinary clinic handbook. Springer-Verlag, New York
Cardenas D D, Larson J, Egan K J 1986 Hysterical paralysis in the upper extremity of chronic pain patients. Archives of Physical Medicine and Rehabilitation 67: 190–193
Caruso L A, Chan D E 1986 Evaluation and management of the patient with acute back pain. American Journal of Occupational Therapy 40: 347–351
Caruso L A, Chan D E, Chan A 1987 The management of work-related back pain. American Journal of Occupational Therapy 41: 112–117
Cronin Mosey A 1974 An alternative: the biopsychosocial model. American Journal of Occupational Therapy 28: 137–140
Cubie S H, Kaplan K 1982 A case analysis method for the model of human occupation. American Journal of Occupational Therapy 36: 645–656
Dolce J J 1987 Self-efficacy and disability beliefs in behavioral treatment of pain. Behaviour Research Therapy 25: 289–299
Dolce J J, Crocker M F, Moletteire C, Doleys D M 1986 Exercise quotas, anticipatory concern and self-efficacy expectancies in chronic pain: a preliminary report. Pain 24: 365–372
Engel G L 1978 The biopsychosocial model and the education of health professionals. Annals of the New York Academy of Science 310: 169–181
Engel G L 1980 The clinical application of the biopsychosocial model. American Journal of Psychiatry 137: 535–544
Engel J M 1990 Commentary on adaptive equipment: its effectiveness for people with chronic lower back pain. Occupational Therapy Journal of Research 10: 122–125
Fishbein M, Ajzen I 1975 Belief, attitude, intention, and behavior. An introduction to theory and research. Addison-Wesley, Reading
Flower A, Naxon E, Jones R E et al 1981 An occupational therapy program for chronic back pain. American Journal of Occupational Therapy 35: 243–248
Gage M 1992 The appraisal model of coping: an assessment and intervention model for occupational therapy. American Journal of Occupational Therapy 46: 353–362
Gage M, Polatajko H J 1994 Enhancing occupational performance through an understanding of perceived self-efficacy. American Journal of Occupational Therapy 48: 452–461
Gage M, Noh S, Polatajko H J, Kaspar V 1994 Measuring perceived self-efficacy in occupational therapy. American Journal of Occupational Therapy 48: 783–790
Galantino M L 1990 Pain management and neuromuscular reeducation for the HIV patient. Occupational Therapy in Health Care 7: 161–170
Giles G M, Allen M E 1986 Occupational therapy in the treatment of the patient with chronic pain. British Journal of Occupational Therapy 49: 4–9
Grant E L 1978 A new dimension to occupational therapy – the pain relief clinic. Proceedings of the 10th Federal Conference of the Australian Association of Occupational Therapists, Sydney
Gusich R L 1984 Occupational therapy for chronic pain: a clinical application of the model of human occupation. Occupational Therapy in Health Care 1: 59–73
Heck S A 1990 Pain management in the acute care setting. American Occupational Therapy Association Newspaper, Occupational Therapy Forum V: 2–4

International Association for the Study of Pain 1993 Directory of Members. IASP, Washington

Jensen M P, Karoly P 1987 Notes on the survey of pain attitudes (SOPA): original (24-item) and revised (35-item) versions. Unpublished manuscript, Arizona State University, Tempe

Jensen M P, Karoly P, Huger R 1987 The development and preliminary validation of an instrument to assess patients' attitudes towards pain. Journal of Psychosomatic Research 31: 393–400

Jensen M P, Turner J A, Romano J M, Karoly P 1991 Coping with chronic pain: a critical review of the literature. Pain 47: 249–283

Johnson J A 1984 Occupational therapy and the patient with pain. Occupational Therapy in Health Care 1: 7–15

Kielhofner G 1980 A model of human occupation, part 3: benign and vicious cycles. American Journal of Occupational Therapy 34: 731–737

Kielhofner G, Burke J P 1980 A model of human occupation, part 1: conceptual framework and content. American Journal of Occupational Therapy 34: 572–581

Kielhofner G, Burke J P, Igi C H 1980 A model of human occupation, part 4: assessment and intervention. American Journal of Occupational Therapy 34: 777–788

Lazarus R A, Folkman S 1984 Stress, appraisal and coping. Springer, New York

Leventhal H, Diefenbach M, Leventhal E A 1992 Illness cognition: using commonsense to understand treatment adherence and affect cognition interactions. Cognitive Therapy and Research 16: 143–163

Lloyd C, Coggles L 1988 Contribution of occupational therapy to pain management in cancer patients with metastatic breast cancer. American Journal of Hospice Care, Nov–Dec: 36–38

McCormack G L 1988 Pain management by occupational therapists. American Journal of Occupational Therapy 42: 582–590

Mangiamele R 1984 In touch with pain: an occupational therapist's perspective. Proceedings of the Australian Association of Occupational Therapists 13th Federal Conference, Perth

Matsutsuyu J 1969 The interest checklist. American Journal of Occupational Therapy 23: 323–328

Matsutsuyu J 1971 Occupational behaviour: a perspective on work and play. American Journal of Occupational Therapy 25: 291–294

Mattingly C 1994 Occupational therapy as a two-body practice: the body as machine. In: Mattingly C, Fleming M H (eds) Clinical reasoning: forms of inquiry in a therapeutic practice. Davis, Philadelphia

Mattingly C, Fleming M H 1994 Giving language to practice. In: Mattingly C, Fleming M H (eds) Clinical reasoning: forms of inquiry in a therapeutic practice. Davis, Philadelphia

Meyer D, Leventhal H, Gutmann M 1985 Common-sense models of illness: the example of hypertension. Health Psychology 4: 115–135

Milne J M 1983 The biopsychosocial model as applied to a multidisciplinary pain management programme. Journal of the New Zealand Association of Occupational Therapists 34: 19–21

Moore N I 1990 The multidisciplinary chronic pain treatment team. In: Miller T W (ed) Chronic pain, volume II. International Universities Press, Connecticut

Moorehead L 1969 The occupational history. The American Journal of Occupational Therapy 23: 329–338

Moss-Morris R, Petrie K 1994 Illness perceptions: implications for occupational therapy. Australian Occupational Therapy Journal 41: 73–82

O'Hara M 1992 Occupational therapy and the pain management team. British Journal of Occupational Therapy 55: 19–20

Pritchard L 1991 The use of groups for relaxation therapy and stress management training as part of a multidisciplinary pain management programme. Proceedings of the 12th Annual Scientific Meeting Australian Pain Society

Riley J F, Ahern D K, Follick M J 1988 Chronic pain and functional impairment: assessing beliefs about their relationship. Archives of Physical Medicine and Rehabilitation 69: 579–582

Rogers J C 1982 Order and disorder in medicine and occupational therapy. American Journal of Occupational Therapy 36: 29–35
Rogers J C 1988 The NPI interest checklist. In: Hemphill B J (ed) Mental health assessment in occupational therapy: an integrative approach to the evaluation process. Slack, Thoroughfare
Schwartz D P, DeGood D E, Shutty M S 1985 Direct assessment of beliefs and attitudes of chronic pain patients. Archives of Physical Medicine and Rehabilitation 66: 806–809
Shutty M S, DeGood D E, Tuttle D H 1990 Chronic pain patients' beliefs about their pain and treatment outcomes. Archives of Physical Medicine and Rehabilitation 71: 128–132
Sikorski J M, Molan R 1987 Task performance and occupational overuse syndromes. Proceedings of the 9th Annual Scientific Meeting Australian Pain Society, Brisbane
Smith M B 1974 Competence and adaptation. American Journal of Occupational Therapy 28: 11–15
Strong J 1984 Occupational therapy services within the pain clinic: a descriptive and evaluative account. Proceedings of the 13th Federal Conference of the Australian Association of Occupational Therapists, Perth
Strong J 1986a Occupational therapy's contribution to pain management in Queensland. Australian Occupational Therapy Journal 33: 101–107
Strong J 1986b Occupational therapy and chronic pain. Proceedings of the 8th Annual Scientific Meeting of the Australian Pain Society, Melbourne
Strong J 1987 Chronic pain management: the occupational therapist's role. British Journal of Occupational Therapy 50: 262–263
Strong J 1989 The occupational therapist's contribution to the management of chronic pain. Patient Management 13: 43–50
Strong J 1990 Commentary response on 'Adaptive equipment: its effectiveness for people with chronic lower back pain'. Occupational Therapy Journal of Research 10: 131–133
Strong J, Ashton R 1992 Psychosocial assessment of the patient with chronic low back pain. Proceedings of the 13th Annual Scientific Meeting of the Australian Pain Society, Perth
Strong J, Ashton R, Cramond T, Chant D 1990 Pain intensity, attitude and function in low back pain patients. Australian Occupational Therapy Journal 37: 179–183
Strong J, Ashton R, Chant D 1992 The measurement of attitudes towards and beliefs about pain. Pain 48: 227–236
Tigges K N, Sherman L M, Sherwin F S 1984 Perspectives on the pain of the hospice patient: the roles of the occupational therapist and physician. Occupational Therapy in Health Care 1: 55–68
Turk D C, Rudy T 1988 A cognitive behavioural perspective on chronic pain: beyond the scalpel and syringe. In: Tollison C D (ed) Handbook of chronic pain management. Williams & Wilkins, Baltimore
Turk D C, Rudy T 1992
Tyson R, Strong J 1990 Adaptive equipment: its effectiveness for people with chronic lower back pain. Occupational Therapy Journal of Research 10: 111–121
Unruh A et al – IASP ad hoc Subcommittee for Occupational Therapy/Physical Therapy Curriculum 1994 Pain curriculum for students in occupational therapy or physical therapy. IASP Newsletter
Vlaeyen J W S, Groenman N H, Thomassen J, Schuerman J A, Van Eek H, Snijders A M J, Van Houten J 1989 A behavioural treatment for sitting and standing intolerance in a patient with chronic low back pain. Clinical Journal of Pain 5: 233–237
Wall P D, Melzack R 1989 Textbook of pain, 2nd edn. Churchill Livingstone, Edinburgh
Wall P D, Melzack R 1994 Textbook of pain, 3rd edn. Churchill Livingstone, Edinburgh
Williams D A, Thorn B E 1989 An empirical assessment of pain beliefs. Pain 36: 351–358
Wynn Parry C B 1982 The 1981 Philip Nichols Memorial Lecture. Internal Rehabilitation Medicine 4: 59–65
Wynn Parry C B 1983 Management of pain in avulsion lesions of the brachial plexus. In: Bonica J J et al Advances in pain research and therapy, vol 5. Raven Press, New York
Wyrick J M, Niemeyer L O, Ellexson M, Jacobs K, Taylor S 1991 Occupational therapy work hardening programs: a demographic study. American Journal of Occupational Therapy 45: 109–112

5

Assessment issues

Why obtain a comprehensive picture of the patient? 71	Biopsychosocial assessment model 78
What do we need to know? 72	The multilevel pain context model 80
The necessary and sufficient dimensions of pain 73	Reliability, validity and sensitivity revisited 81
Measurement of perceptions of pain 73	What does the occupational therapist measure? 82
The integrated psychosocial assessment model 75	Performance system 82
Some assessment models 76	Habituation system 82
The West Haven Yale multidimensional pain inventory 77	Volitional system 85
	Self-efficacy measurement 87
Integrated pain assessment model 78	Case example 87
	Chapter summary 89
	References 90

Assessment of clinical pain is a difficult multidimensional problem for clinicians. Whether the objective is to obtain descriptions of the individual patient's pain experience or to measure changes in pain perception after treatment, reliable and valid instrumentation is necessary (Burkhardt 1984).

In this chapter I will explain why I consider a comprehensive assessment of the patient with pain to be essential practice for the occupational therapist working in this area. Current thinking on the need for a detailed assessment is described. This is followed by an examination of the necessary and sufficient dimensions required to assess a multidimensional phenomenon like pain. A number of assessment models will then be outlined. Of course, any consideration of assessment is never complete without reference to the notions of reliability, validity and sensitivity, and these issues are also briefly mentioned.

This chapter does not pretend to be a textbook on pain assessment; yet a book on occupational therapy and pain would be incomplete without a discussion, albeit brief, on pain assessment. If, at the end of the chapter, the reader wants to pursue the matter of pain assessment further (and hopefully he will), he is referred to the seminal works on pain assessment, beginning with Beecher (1957) and continuing with Chapman et al (1985), Karoly and Jensen (1987) and Turk and Melzack (1992).

WHY OBTAIN A COMPREHENSIVE PICTURE OF THE PATIENT?

It is a widely held belief that sound clinical intervention needs to be based on thorough assessment practice, irrespective of the disorder being treated, and this is equally true with the condition of chronic pain. The Australian National Health and Medical Research Council (1988) stated that: 'it [pain measurement] needs to be further developed and more widely applied'.

Two possible problems can be identified in current pain assessment practice. First, the field of pain assessment and measurement remains in its infancy. Chapman and his colleagues (1985) attributed the lack of progress in pain measurement to the inherently complex nature of the pain experience. Secondly, since pain is a multidimensional phenomenon, there is a need to measure the multiple dimensions. However, it must first be decided exactly what these dimensions are. The words of Karoly (1985) remain pertinent: 'Although it is probably obvious that unidimensional, one-shot, atheoretical approaches to pain measurement provide little worthwhile data to the assessor, the exact formulas for "comprehensive", "integrated", "multimodal", "interactional", "multifaceted", or "broadbanded" assessment programs have not been readily forthcoming.'

What do we need to know?

It is my contention that, to provide a good service to our patients and clients, we must first gain a comprehensive picture of them, and of their strengths and weaknesses. In Chapter 4, I stated that I do not follow the strictly behaviourist view, which holds that to focus on the patient's pain is to reinforce it. If I am to work with a patient with pain, as I very often do, then I need to understand a whole host of things about that patient – such as, what sort of pain they have, what happens to the pain when they sit or stand or 'do', how does the pain interfere with their occupation, their goals and their dreams? If I cannot or do not draw such a picture, then I contend that my therapy will not be focused. In fact, my therapy runs the risk of being of little value. Certainly, there are often generic therapy components which we probably do not need an elaborate assessment to determine. For example, the individual with tension contraction headache pain may benefit from relaxation training, or the person with low back pain may benefit from education in correct body mechanics and back care. But even these components need to be refined for different people. For example, a patient with no ability to visualize images will derive little benefit from relaxation based upon imagery, and a woman with a small baby may need very different back care advice from that suited to a woman in a sedentary occupation or a man in a manual job.

Time spent by the occupational therapist in conducting a thorough assessment will be rewarded by more efficacious therapy and a better therapeutic relationship. Other writers too have stressed the importance of the comprehensive assessment of the patient with pain. A comprehensive, multidimensional assessment must be made of the patient with chronic pain in order to understand the problems faced by the patient, to make an accurate diagnosis, to design an optimal treatment program, to evaluate the effectiveness of that treatment program, and to increase our understanding of pain mechanisms (Chapman et al 1985, Karoly 1985).

THE NECESSARY AND SUFFICIENT DIMENSIONS OF PAIN

We really do not know what clinical pain is; at present, even the number and the characteristics of the dimensions are in dispute. Clearly, the first step toward quantification of pain is a better understanding of its dimensions (Clark et al 1989).

When considering the number of dimensions to assess in the pain patient, it is clear that while there are some similar thoughts, there is no clear consensus in the literature. Many researchers and clinicians recommend a trimodal approach to the assessment of the pain patient. But should this approach encompass the sensory, affective and evaluative dimensions suggested by Melzack (1975), or the subjective, behavioural and physiological dimensions proposed by Grabois and Blacker (1987) and McGrath and Unruh (1987)? Or yet again, should the approach be the integrated assessment of psychosocial, behavioural and biomedical dimensions as suggested by Turk and his colleagues (Kerns et al 1985, Turk & Rudy 1987, 1988)?

What are the dimensions of pain, what are the patients' perceptions of their experience of pain, and how should the clinician/researcher go about measuring such variables? A useful place to start may well be to ask the patients. When we turn to the literature, however, we find that there have been few documented studies of patients' perceptions of living with pain. Interestingly, much of this available literature comes from the 1970s and 1980s. Perhaps in this technologically focused decade, patients' perceptions have been relegated to the background while our preoccupation with objectivity has come to the foreground. The words of Melzack and Torgerson (1971) still apply: 'Few studies have attempted to specify the dimensions of pain experience'.

Five aspects of the pain experience of prime importance to occupational therapists working in the area are those suggested by Turk and Kerns (1983); these are listed in Box 5.1.

Measurement of perceptions of pain

The importance of assessing the patient's perception of his pain has been acknowledged by Turk and his colleagues (Kerns et al 1985, Turk & Kerns 1983, Turk & Rudy 1987). There has, however, been little attention paid to

> **Box 5.1** The five dimensions of the pain experience
>
> Turk and Kerns (1983) suggested that the five dimensions of the pain experience which need to be assessed are:
>
> 1. descriptive characteristics of pain
> 2. the patient's perception of pain
> 3. physical, cognitive and behavioural responses to pain
> 4. the impact of pain on the patient's life
> 5. coping mechanisms used to deal with the pain.

the measurement of such a dimension. Very often in the clinical and research setting, the patient's perceptions of the pain experience have been confined to self-reporting on selected aspects such as pain intensity, location and quality (Keefe 1987) using questionnaires such as the McGill Pain Questionnaire (Melzack 1975) and the Visual Analogue Scale (Scott & Huskisson 1979) or, more recently, on dimensions such as attitudes and coping, using questionnaires such as the Survey of Pain Attitudes (Jensen et al 1987) and the Coping Strategy Questionnaire (Rosenstiel & Keefe 1983). That is to say, the patient's self-reporting is often constrained by preconceived ideas imposed by the researcher/clinician via the medium of a printed questionnaire.

Melzack and Torgerson (1971) examined the dimensions of pain as measured by pain descriptors. A priori development of a list of 102 words was made on the basis of an examination of the clinical pain literature and earlier lists. The McGill Pain Questionnaire (Melzack 1975) was based on the findings from these studies by Melzack and Torgerson.

Moore (1990), in acknowledging the possible a priori biases of researchers in examining pain coping strategies, had subjects generate responses to a set of questions on types of dental pain and ways to relieve such pain. Items for use in further investigation were derived from a content analysis of subject responses. Similarly, when looking at beliefs about pain, Williams and Thorn (1989) asked back pain subjects to describe the beliefs they had about their pain condition; seven belief content areas were thus derived. These beliefs were about:

- when the pain would cease
- whether the pain was constant or intermittent
- the cause of the pain
- the mysterious nature of pain
- how pain impacts upon one's lifestyle
- personal pain control
- blame for pain.

We (Strong et al 1994a) recently explored the necessary and sufficient dimensions of chronic back pain as seen through the eyes of individuals with pain. Guided by the words of Clark et al (1989) – '... the investigator must put aside his preconceptions and allow the patient to inform him' – we adopted a qualitative approach to this endeavour. The results of this study will be briefly considered here.

Seven patients (four women and three men) with chronic low back pain participated in the study. The subjects were representative examples of patients seen at the pain clinic. They had extensive and well documented histories of chronic low back pain. The participants had an average age of 58.43 years (S.D. = 11.13). In comparison with other large chronic low back pain samples, such as the one used by Strong et al (1991) the patients were significantly older (t = 2.34, $p<.05$), had been in pain for significantly more years (t = 2.14, $p<.05$), and had undergone significantly more pain-related operations (t = 2.97, $p<.01$). It could be safely presumed then, that the selected subjects were well qualified to discuss what it was like to live with chronic low back pain.

The findings from the focus groups conducted with these patients provided some useful clues for deciding what to include in a comprehensive multidimensional assessment. From the patients' perspectives, the themes of family/personal relationships, positive and negative affect/emotions, symptoms/features of pain, mobility, domestic activities and treatment were important (Strong et al 1994a).

The integrated psychosocial assessment model

We have now considered the dimensions considered important by individuals with pain who participated in our study. It is also important to consider the perspectives of experts in the area of pain management. As I said (Strong 1992a) 'No picture of the dimensions of chronic low back pain can be complete without the input gained from the health care professional working in the area'. Based on a survey conducted with health professionals who were members of the Australian Pain Society, a review of the literature and the integration of the patients' perspectives, an assessment model with the dimensions listed below was identified.

The model posits that assessment needs to be made of the dimensions of:

- pain intensity
- pain location/extent
- functional status
- attitudes towards and beliefs about pain
- coping strategies
- depression
- illness behaviour.

76 OCCUPATIONAL THERAPY CONCERNS

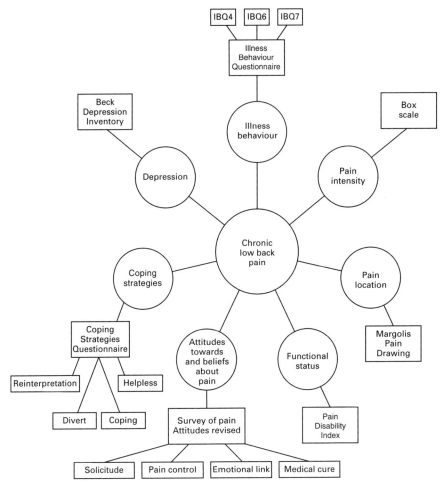

Figure 5.1 Working psychosocial assessment model for the patient with chronic low back pain. (Adapted from Strong et al 1995, with permission.)

This assessment model, the Integrated Psychosocial Assessment Model (Strong et al 1994b) is illustrated in Figure 5.1.

SOME ASSESSMENT MODELS

In this section, four comprehensive assessment models for use with patients with chronic pain will be considered.

The West Haven Yale Multidimensional Pain Inventory (WHYMPI) (Kerns et al 1985) was developed as a comprehensive measure of not only such things as pain severity, but also the patient's appraisals of how pain interferes with his life, and the amount of support given by significant others (Turk & Rudy 1988). While suggesting that a trimodal assessment of chronic pain is essential, Turk and his colleagues advocated an *integrated* multidimensional assessment of the psychosocial, behavioural and biomedical dimensions of a person's pain (Kerns et al 1985, Rudy et al 1990, Turk & Rudy 1987, 1988). More recently, the Medical Examination and Diagnostic Information Coding System (MEDICS) was published, which assesses the biomedical dimension (Rudy et al 1990). This model attempts to integrate the various pieces of psychosocial and behavioural data into a comprehensive assessment. Later work has concentrated on defining and refining a comprehensive assessment for the biomedical dimension.

The West Haven Yale multidimensional pain inventory

The WHYMPI, or the MPI as it is frequently referred to, was developed on the basis of the cognitive behavioural theory of pain management (Kerns et al 1985). A three-part inventory, it measures:

- interference caused by pain
- support received
- severity of pain
- perceived self-control
- negative mood
- punishing responses of others
- solicitous responses of others
- distracting responses of others
- frequency with which activities (household, outdoor, social and away from home) are performed.

Using the MPI, Turk and Rudy (1987, 1988) were able to identify three distinct patient subgroups. These three groups were:

1. 'dysfunctional' patients (42.6% of sample)
2. 'interpersonally distressed' patients (27.9% of sample)
3. 'minimizers/adaptive copers' (29.5% of sample).

When the biomedical data were integrated with the WHYMPI data, four distinct patient clusters were found (Turk & Rudy 1987, 1988):

1. 'disabled' (24% of sample)
2. 'dysfunctional' (24% of sample)
3. 'interpersonally distressed' (31% of sample)
4. 'minimizers/adaptive copers' (21% of sample).

The possible clinical utility of this assessment model is great. Such an assessment model may assist clinicians in designing treatment programs which suit individual patient characteristics (Turk & Rudy 1988). This assessment model is to be commended for its attempt to deal with multiple data in a multidimensional way (Vlaeyen et al 1989). It also, quite clearly, has provided tools to measure these three dimensions. Numerous studies now include the WHYMPI as a measurement tool.

Integrated pain assessment model

We have also developed a multidimensional assessment model which has been used, thus far, with patients with chronic low back pain (Strong et al 1994b). This integrated Pain Assessment Model (IPAM) contains the dimensions of the patient's pain intensity, functional ability/disability, attitudes towards and beliefs about pain, coping strategies, depression and illness behaviour.

Cluster analysis of the IPAM data from 100 patients with chronic low back pain attending hospital pain clinics or neurosurgical units in Brisbane, Australia revealed the presence of three distinct patient sub-groups:

1. *In control patients* (n = 48). These patients had low pain intensity, low use of diverting and helpless coping strategies, and a strong belief that they could control their pain.

2. *Depressed and disabled patients* (n = 23). These patients had high disability, high depression, high use of helpless coping strategies, high irritability, and high beliefs in solicitude and an emotional link to their pain.

3. *Active coping patients with high denial* (n = 29). These patients reported using multiple coping strategies, but continued to have high pain intensity and a high denial score.

We showed the validity of this clustering solution by an examination of variables external to the clustering solution.

In a further study on the IPAM with patients seen at the Auckland Regional Pain Service, we conducted a replication of this clustering model using an independent sample of 70 patients with chronic low back pain. Data analysis supports the existence of these same three clusters (Strong et al 1995).

Biopsychosocial assessment model

Another assessment approach is the biopsychosocial approach of Waddell and his colleagues, developed specifically for patients with chronic low back pain (Waddell 1987, Waddell et al 1984a, 1984b). A biopsychosocial illness model rather than a disease model is advocated, with consideration given to the physical, psychological and social elements (Waddell et al 1984b). The model is illustrated in Figure 5.2.

Using this model, Waddell and his co-workers have illustrated the distinction (or desynchrony) between pain and disability, and between illness behaviour, distress and signs of physical disease (Waddell & Main 1984). Work has focused on the development and refinement of measurement tools to tap some of these areas. For example, the Chronic Disability Index (Waddell 1987, Waddell & Main 1984), the Modified Somatic Perceptions Questionnaire (Main 1983), and the Waddell Impairment Index (Waddell & Main 1984) have been developed.

The biopsychosocial assessment model thus takes a number of steps forward: it focuses on one specific type of chronic pain, and it has considered the properties of measurement tools designed to tap some of the relevant areas. However, the model does not appear to make explicit why these specific dimensions or variables were chosen to the exclusion of others. Furthermore, no formal mechanism for the integration of data has

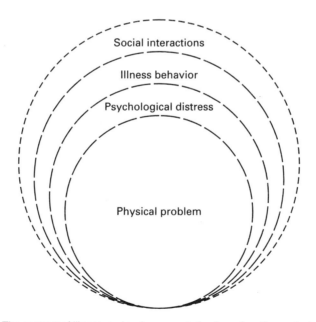

Figure 5.2 The concept of illness: a visual representation based on the analysis of disability in chronic low back pain. (Adapted from Waddell & Main 1984, with permission.)

been published, apart from correlations obtained between some of the variables and the use of multiple regression statistical procedures.

The multilevel pain context model

The Multilevel Pain Context Model (Karoly 1985, Karoly & Jensen 1987) posits that the fundamental unit of analysis should be an interactional one comprising the patient in pain and 'his or her social and inanimate environments' (Karoly 1985). A number of contexts or dimensions simultaneously contribute to the pain phenomenon. These contexts are:

- biomedical (why does the patient hurt?)
- focal/experiential (as experienced by the patient)
- meaning/relational (what difference does the pain make?)
- conceptual/sociological (what is the overriding philosophy of the assessor, or treatment facility?).

The model asserts that all contexts should be considered together, not in isolation. In particular, it urges against the mind–body dichotomy, which for too long has hampered our understanding, assessment and subsequent treatment of patients with chronic pain. This dualistic and limiting thinking remains in effect in some quarters, as shown by the recent words of a patient with chronic low back pain of 11 years' duration: 'Everybody said, they looked at me and said, you know, "You're crazy". I was sent to psychiatrists and everything else and the psychiatrist sort of came back with the answer, "It's not up here, the problem's not there. You're not crazy as such" ' (Strong 1992a).

This model has provided an overview of various pain measurement tools which are available for the first three levels of pain (that is, the biomedical, focal and meaning levels), as well as some studies of the properties of some of these instruments (Jensen et al 1986, 1987, Karoly & Jensen 1987).

Karoly and Jensen (1987) have provided a conceptual framework for the integration of data from this multilevel assessment. The likelihood of desynchrony within the focal/experiential dimension is raised. It is suggested that integration of data should be guided by a consideration of the patient's pain problem 'within the related frameworks of time, place and meaning'. Clinicians may consider using this as a heuristic tool; it does not constitute a set of postulates which can be subjected to empirical scrutiny.

At the moment, the Pain Context Model (Karoly 1985) stands as an assessment model of promise. It has been developed across all types of chronic pain patients, rather than for a specific diagnostic group. However, like the other models, it has received minimal examination. In addition, it lacks a method for the actual integration of data from the various sources.

RELIABILITY, VALIDITY AND SENSITIVITY REVISITED

Now that a number of assessment models have been identified, it is necessary to find the most reliable and valid methods for the measurement of each dimension of the model. For an excellent analysis of issues related to measurement standards, the interested reader is referred to the paper by Johnstone and his colleagues (1992). These important issues are examined briefly below.

Validity

Validity considers whether a test measures what it purports to measure (Johnstone et al 1992, Lindeman & Merenda 1979). Thinking of an individual with pain, we might ask if a measure of functioning, such as lifting a weight from knee-height to shoulder-height, might also be measuring the person's beliefs about what movement will cause them pain, or may 'break' their fusion. Types of validity to be considered include face validity, content validity, construct validity, and criterion-related validity (Lindeman & Merenda 1979). The sensitivity of the measurement tool is a part of criterion-related validity. This refers to the ability of the test to detect real changes which occur over time, and real differences which exist between patients.

Reliability

Reliability refers to the consistency with which an assessment tool measures the particular phenomenon of interest (Lindeman & Merenda 1979). With respect to the pain area, if the scoring system of a functional status scale is open to interpretation, then the scoring of the same patient by two different occupational therapists may yield different results. For example, if a scale uses as outcomes only the words 'good outcome', 'fair outcome', and 'poor outcome', one occupational therapist may rate a patient who returns to performing all personal activities of daily living (ADLs) as having a good recovery, while another occupational therapist may rate that patient's outcome as only fair, since they still have not returned to work.

Utility

The utility of the measurement tool also needs to be considered. Utility is concerned with how usable the tool is. Does it take too long to administer, is it too complex to score, or is the apparatus required too expensive for the facility's budget? With respect to the pain area, for example, a questionnaire which takes 30 minutes to complete will probably not be appropriate for use with a patient with pain from terminal cancer.

WHAT DOES THE OCCUPATIONAL THERAPIST MEASURE?

In many settings, the occupational therapist works with patients with pain as part of a broader team. In such situations, the comprehensive assessment of the patient will be made by the team as a whole. Not every team member will need to assess all dimensions, since this would be unwieldy and tedious for both the patient and the team. The most important thing is for a complete picture to be developed and shared across the team. However, there may be situations where the occupational therapist does not have the luxury of working within a dedicated team, for example, when a person with pain is referred to the regional hospital for occupational therapy assistance, or when the consulting occupational therapist to a nursing home discovers a resident with chronic pain. In these types of situation, the occupational therapist will need to spend time carefully building a picture of that patient's pain.

In an existing multidisciplinary team, what assessments would I, as the occupational therapist, usually perform? How would the assessment tasks be divided up amongst the team members?

In considering which areas of assessment the occupational therapist would be concerned with, it is useful to refer back to my occupational therapy practice model synthesized in Chapter 4. I am generally concerned with the patient's performance, habituation and volitional systems. A summary of some of the assessments which may be used for each of these systems is given in Box 5.2.

Performance system

Starting with the performance system, my assessment may consider the areas of self-care, work, rest, and play. Assessment of instrumental activities of daily living (IADLs), personal activities of daily living (PADLs), work, strength, range of motion and sensation may be relevant here. The functional status of patients is frequently assessed using measures such as the Pain Disability Index (Pollard 1985, Tait et al 1987, Tait et al 1990) or the Oswestry Low Back Pain Disability Index (Fairbank et al 1980). Aspects of mobility such as sitting and standing tolerances are typically assessed by questionnaires such as the Oswestry, used in combination with observation. A comprehensive discussion of the performance components of functioning and work in Chapter 6 will expand on the types of assessments which can be used for this area.

Habituation system

With respect to the habituation system of the patient, the occupational therapist needs to consider the current, past and future roles of the

> **Box 5.2** Assessments which can be used for comprehensive assessment of the patient with pain
>
> *Performance system**
> Functional status   Pain Disability Index (Tait et al 1987)
>   Oswestry Low Back Pain Disability Index (Fairbank et al 1980)
>
> *Habituation system*
> Roles and habits   Interview
>   24-hour log (Larrington 1970)
>   Occupational History (Moorehead 1969, Kielhofner et al 1986)
>   Role Checklist (Oakley 1982, cited in Barris et al 1988)
>   Activity Diary (Fordyce et al 1984)
>   Occupational Performance History Interview (Kielhofner et al 1988a, 1988b)
>
> *Volitional system*
>   NPI Interest Checklist (Matsutsuyu 1969)
>   Survey of Pain Attitudes Revised (Jensen et al 1987)
>   Pain beliefs and Perceptions Inventory (Williams & Thorn 1989)
>   Movement and Pain Prediction Scale (Council et al 1988)
>   Self-Efficacy Gauge (Gage et al 1994)
>   Pain Self-Efficacy Questionnaire (Nicholas 1994)
>
> * See Chapter 6 for further coverage of the assessment of performance components of work, self-care, rest and leisure

individual. Let us reconsider the case of Mrs P, which we looked at in Chapter 4 (Box 4.3). You will recall that Mrs P was a 50-year-old woman with a 12-year history of post-herpetic neuralgia. Her previous life roles had included paid worker (cook), wife and homemaker. Her current role consisted of being an invalid and a pain patient. In discussions with her occupational therapist, she determined that a desired future life role was to be a good spouse and homemaker again. Note that her desired life role was not contingent upon being 'a pain-free person'. This successful separation of pain and pain relief from life roles is an important part of the rehabilitation process which the occupational therapist encourages.

Useful tools for the therapist

With respect to the measurement of a patient's roles and habits, the occupational therapist has at her fingertips a number of useful tools, including an unstructured or semistructured interview, the 24-hour log (Larrington 1970), the occupational history (Moorehead 1969), the role checklist (Barris et al 1988) and the activity diary (Fordyce et al 1984).

The 24-hour log. The 24-hour log (Larrington 1970) can be used to record the content of a person's time, recorded in 15-minute intervals. The log also elicits information on whether the individual would want more or less of a particular activity, whether it was a solo or cooperative activity, and whether it was a special or a routine activity. The log was developed to be used in conjunction with an unstructured interview (Larrington 1970). Larrington reported that an interview based on the log completion was more sensitive and yielded more valid answers than a more general interview.

The occupational history. This is a tool yielding information on the individual's history, which helps the occupational therapist to understand both 'the functional deficits and strengths' of patients (Moorehead 1969). Further developments in the assessment of occupational history have been made by a number of workers:

- Florey and Michelman (1982) developed the occupational role screening interview, for use with patients with psychiatric disabilities. This interview examined 23 matters related to worker/homemaker roles, along with 11 questions about school. The interview enables the occupational therapist to obtain a synthesized picture of the status of the individual's role function and the balance between occupation and leisure (Florey & Michelman 1982). At the time of its publication (1982), the authors reported that work on its reliability and predictive capacity was underway.
- Kielhofner and his colleagues (1986) developed the occupational role history, for use with clients with physical disabilities. It contains 11 pairs of items representative of parts of the model of human occupation. Each item is scored on a 1–5 scale, where 1 = highly dysfunctional and 5 = highly functional (Kielhofner et al 1986). Item intraclass coefficients for inter-rater reliability ranged from 0.38 to 0.93, while Pearson's **r** correlation coefficients for test–retest reliability ranged from 0.61 to 0.96. It was reported that four items had less than moderate inter-rater reliability and one item was unsatisfactory for test–retest reliability (Kielhofner et al 1986).
- Kielhofner and Henry (1988a, 1988b) developed the occupational performance history interview. It contains 39 questions concerning the areas of environmental factors, life roles, organization of daily routines, perceptions of ability and responsibility, and values, interests and goals (Kielhofner & Henry 1988). A 5-point scale is used to score the individual's function in each of the five areas, where 1 = totally maladaptive and 5 = totally adaptive. Test–retest reliabilities of 0.31–0.68 were reported for individual items of the interview (Pearson's **r** correlations). Inter-rater reliabilities of –0.08–0.55 were obtained. Its authors pointed out that variability may exist where therapists are operating with different frames of reference (Kielhofner & Henry 1988b). It was found to have clinical utility (although it takes about 90 minutes to complete) (Kielhofner & Henry 1988b). Lynch and Bridle (1993) have examined the construct validity of the occupational performance history interview when used

with 143 individuals with spinal cord injury. Support was given to its construct validity by the association of poorer occupational performance in those individuals with greater pain and depression (Lynch & Bridle 1993).

Activity diary. An activity diary can be used by individuals with pain to monitor their activity type and duration (Fordyce et al 1984, Keefe & Dolan 1986, Sanders 1983). For each time period of 1 hour (or 30 minutes), individuals also record their pain intensity level and their medication intake. A sample diary form is contained in the paper by Fordyce et al (1984). Follick and his colleagues (1984) have examined the reliability and validity of the activity diary used with patients with pain. Significant correlations were found between patient and spouse reports for time spent lying down and standing/walking and pain rating. Patients' ratings within and across categories of activities were found to be statistically reliable. A high correlation was also found between the patient's report of downtime and an electromechanical measure of downtime. Support was thus given to the activity diary's reliability and validity (Follick et al 1984).

Role checklist. The role checklist is a two-part instrument which measures roles in an individual's life and the importance of such roles to the individual (Oakley 1982, cited in Barris et al 1988). It has been well described in Barris et al (1988), and is contained as an appendix in Hemphill (1988). Test–retest reliability examination using both percentage agreement and kappa coefficients indicated mostly moderate to substantial agreement for role participation, with slightly lower agreement for the value of activity section (Barris et al 1988). No work on the checklist's concurrent validity (Barris et al 1988) or construct validity has been reported. The tool has, however, good clinical utility.

Volitional system

Assessment of the individual's volitional system can include an examination of his interests (past, current and future), his goals (past, current and future), his attitudes, beliefs, appraisals and coping strategies, and his affective status, self-esteem and self-efficacy. Measurement tools may include the:

- NPI Interest Checklist (Matsutsuyu 1969)
- Survey of Pain Attitudes Revised (Jensen et al 1987, Jensen & Karoly 1987)
- Pain Beliefs and Perceptions Inventory (Williams & Thorn 1989)
- Movement and Pain Perceptions Scale (Council et al 1988)
- Self-Efficacy Gauge (Gage et al 1994)
- Pain Self-Efficacy Questionnaire (Nicholas 1994).

Turk and Melzack (1992) examine a plethora of assessment tools which can be used for different aspects of this dimension. Here, we review a few measures which the occupational therapist may find useful.

Useful tools for the therapist

NPI interest checklist. The Neuropsychiatric Institute (NPI) Interest Checklist (Matsutsuyu 1969) was developed to gather information on the types of, and intensity of, interests held by individuals. It also taps the ability of respondents to express preferences and to discriminate between intensity and type of interest (Matsutsuyu 1969). The checklist contains 80 items of possible interest to which respondents indicate casual, strong or no interest. It yields data on five categories of interest, these being activities of daily living, manual skills, cultural/educational activities, physical sports and social recreation. Matsutsuyu (1969) said of the measure: 'Its limitation is that it is not a test meeting the rigid requirements of psychometric testing'. Rogers (1988) reviewed the properties of the NPI Checklist. She cited a 1979 study by Weinstein which found an overall reliability coefficient for test–retest reliability of 0.92. In discussing the content validity of the checklist, Rogers pointed out that the items had been developed for the particular setting, and as such, its content validity for other settings must be carefully considered. No work on its construct validity has been undertaken. Rogers (1988) considered that: 'Appraisal of the reliability and validity of the NPI Interest Checklist is a high priority for research'.

Survey of pain attitudes revised (SOPAR), and pain beliefs and perceptions inventory (PBPI). In 1992, we reviewed four available tests used to measure patients' attitudes towards and beliefs about their pain and its measurement (Strong et al 1992). We then examined the psychometric properties of two of these measures, the SOPAR and the PBPI. We found good support for the SOPAR in terms of its reliability and validity. The six subscales of the SOPAR had Cronbach's alpha values ranging from 0.49–0.84. A factor analysis on our data from 100 patients indicated the presence of six factors similar to those reported by Jensen et al (1987). Expected correlations between the SOPAR subscales and the Coping Strategy Questionnaire provided support for the construct validity of the SOPAR. Our findings on the PBPI were less supportive. While the internal consistency of the three subscales was reasonable (ranging from 0.67–0.78), no support was found for the construct validity of the scales. Nor was the three-factor structure replicated. Instead, we suggested that the PBPI was tapping four rather than three scales. More recent work by Herda et al (1994) in Germany, Williams et al (1994) in the USA, and Morley and Wilkinson (1995) in Britain has replicated our findings of a four-factor structure for the PBPI.

Self-efficacy measurement

Bandura (1982) has described self-efficacy as 'concerned with judgements of how well one can execute courses of action required to deal with prospective situations'. This concept of self-efficacy is an important one for occupational therapists to consider when working with patients with pain. In 1992 I commented that 'If you can show me that I can achieve something here and now, then yes, I'm much more likely to think I can do it when I leave the clinic' (Strong 1992b). There are three self-efficacy measures which have been used with patients with pain.

Movement and pain perceptions scale (MAPPS). The MAPPS examines the respondent's perceived ability to perform 10 simple movements to completion (for example, bending to touch the toes) (Council et al 1988). Expected pain levels for each step of the movement and reasons for not being able to complete the movement are also elicited. Movement predictions are scored on a 5-point scale, where 1 = unable to perform any stage of the movement, and 5 = able to successfully perform the complete movement (Council et al 1988). No psychometric properties on the MAPPS were reported in this article by Council and his colleagues. I recently found an alpha coefficient of 0.90 indicating good internal consistency for the MAPPS (Strong 1995).

Pain self-efficacy questionnaire (PSEQ). The PSEQ is a 10-item questionnaire containing items felt to typify a variety of activities which patients with chronic pain have difficulty performing (Nicholas 1994). Patients are asked to rate how confident they are about doing each activity despite the pain, using a scale where 0 = not at all confident and 6 = completely confident (Nicholas 1994). The PSEQ has good internal consistency (alpha coefficient of 0.92), good test–retest reliability ($r = 0.79$), and good concurrent and construct validity. It is also sensitive to treatment changes.

Self-efficacy gauge. The Self-Efficacy Gauge (Gage et al 1994) contains 27 activities rated on a 10-point scale, where 1 = not at all confident and 10 = completely confident. Test–retest reliability yielded an intraclass correlation coefficient of 0.90. A Cronbach's alpha value of 0.94 provided support for internal consistency. Support for convergent validity was provided by a significant negative correlation with hopelessness and a positive significant correlation with actual performance of the activities (Gage et al 1994).

CASE EXAMPLE

The case example in Box 5.3 gives an overview of an assessment completed by an occupational therapist of a 58-year-old woman who pre-

88 OCCUPATIONAL THERAPY CONCERNS

Box 5.3 The case of Mrs K

Medical history

Mrs K, a 58-year-old woman developed low back pain and left-sided sciatica following a lifting injury at home 4 years prior to this hospitalization. 2 years ago, she had an L5–S1 disc excision. On this second presentation to hospital, she had low back pain with left-sided sciatica with radiation to the left buttock and left posterior thigh and posterolateral calf with radiation toward the ankle. There was an associated poorly localized paraesthesia in the calf and foot. Myelogram findings provided no significant evidence of disc protrusion.

Assessment

Performance system
Pain intensity. 8/10 on the Box Scale, where 0 = no pain, and 10 = worst possible pain. This was a high self-report of pain.
Functional ability/disability. Pain Disability Index – 25/70. This was a low score.
Pain description. Words chosen on the McGill Pain Questionnaire (Melzack 1975) were burning, stinging, aching, miserable, radiating and drawing.

Volitional system
Survey of Pain Attitudes Revised (SOPAR)
SOPAR Solicitude 16/24
SOPAR Medical cure 22/24
SOPAR Emotional link 15/24
SOPAR Disability 5/16
SOPAR Medication 12/16
SOPAR Pain control 11/36.
These scores indicated a high belief in a medical cure, a belief that medication would help her pain, a need for solicitude and support, yet low disability from the pain. She also had a low belief that she could do anything to help control her pain.

Coping Strategy Questionnaire (CSQ)
CSQ Diverting attention 16/36
CSQ Reinterpreting pain sensations 8/36
CSQ Catastrophizing 14/36
CSQ Ignoring sensations 17/36
CSQ Praying/hoping 23/36
CSQ Coping self-statements 21/36
CSQ Increased behavioural activities 24/36
CSQ Pain control 3/6
CSQ Pain decrease 3/6.

Beck Depression Inventory (Beck et al 1961) 10/63. Kerns and Haythornthwaite (1988) suggest that a score between 0 and 9 indicates no depression, a score between 10 and 17 indicates mild depression, and a score greater than or equal to 18 indicates depression. Using these criteria, Mrs K might have been mildly depressed.

Illness Behaviour Questionnaire (IBQ). IBQ Denial 3 [as compared to an Adelaide General Practice sample mean score of 2.91, and an Adelaide Pain Clinic sample mean score of 3.88 (Pilowsky & Spence 1983)].

Self-efficacy MAPPS. 18/40, where 0 = ability to move without limitation, and 40 = total inability to do the movements. She reported all movements to be limited by pain.

Habituation system
Occupational roles. Married, lived in own home with husband. Was the primary homemaker. She had two grown children, both daughters, who were married and lived locally.

> **Box 5.3** cont'd
>
> *Interests.* She reported few interests. She and her husband had a hobby farm, but she found it difficult to sit for the long drive to the farm at weekends.
>
> **Assessment summary**
>
> Mrs K described herself as having a minimal level of dysfunction due to the pain. Yet she reported a high level of pain. She was independent in all areas of ADL, particularly personal ADLs. It was in the areas of social activities and recreation that Mrs K expressed some limitations. Her physical mobility was fairly good, yet she did not perform some movements due to her fear of pain. She could sit for an hour without distress, and could stand for around 30 minutes.
>
> Mrs K had a firm belief in a medical cure for her pain. She thought that medication would help her. She had a strong desire for solicitude, and a low belief in her own ability to manage her pain. She reported using many strategies to try and cope with her pain. She denied having any underlying problems – if it were not for her pain, all in her life would be fine. Her denial score was higher than for a sample of patients attending general practice facilities, but lower than a pain clinic sample.
>
> In terms of life roles, now that her two daughters had married and left home, it seemed that Mrs K felt some sense of loss and rolelessness. It could be that Mrs K experienced pain more intensely due to her feelings of loss. It may be that the pain was a legitimate way to get attention and help. Such somatization of an emotional state is a frequently seen occurrence. The sum of these findings suggest that Mrs K might have been somatizing. She reported a high level of pain, for which she wanted medical help and support from her loved ones. Yet she was not particularly disabled by her pain. She felt she had little control over her pain. She had some role losses in her life, but denied she had any personal/emotional problems. Now that a comprehensive assessment had been made of Mrs K, her pain, her functioning, her volition and her habituation, a management program which addressed her individual needs could be developed and implemented.

sented for management of chronic low back pain. While the three systems of the model of human occupation are considered (see p. 58), the integrated psychosocial assessment model (see p. 75) is also used in the assessment process.

CHAPTER SUMMARY

This chapter explained why it is so necessary for the occupational therapist to undertake a thorough assessment of the individual with pain, and suggested the necessary and sufficient dimensions to consider in such a comprehensive assessment. A number of integrated models were then presented, including our own integrated psychosocial assessment model. At the risk of sounding like a cracked record (or perhaps worse, a statistics lecture), I then reviewed what we mean by the terms reliability, validity and utility. Then, the assessment areas of concern to an occupational therapist were considered, using the framework offered by the model of human occupation. Box 5.2 summarizes the various assessments which can be used to assess the three different subsystems of the individual patient's life that are highlighted in the model of human occupation. Finally, a complete example of an occupational therapy assessment of a patient with chronic pain was given. This example illustrates why I believe a comprehensive assessment of the individual with pain is so necessary.

In Chapter 6, we progress to the area of treatment or management, and begin to look at occupational therapy management practices, using as a framework the guiding concepts of activities of daily living, work, rest and play.

REFERENCES

Bandura A 1982 Self-efficacy mechanisms in human agency. American Psychologist 37: 122–147

Barris R, Oakley F, Kielhofner G 1988 The role checklist. In: Hemphill B J (ed) Mental health assessment in occupational therapy: an integrative approach to the evaluation process. Slack, Thoroughfare

Beck A T, Ward C H, Mendelson M, Mock J, Erbauch J 1961 An inventory for measuring depression. Archives of General Psychiatry 4: 561–571

Beecher H K 1957 The measurement of pain. Pharmacological Reviews 9: 56–209

Burckhardt C S 1984 The use of the McGill pain questionnaire in assessing arthritis pain. Pain 19: 305–314

Chapman C R, Casey K L, Dubner R, Foley K M, Gracely R H, Reading A E 1985 Pain measurement: an overview. Pain 22: 1–31

Clark W C, Janel M N, Carroll J D 1989 Multidimensional pain requires multidimensional scaling. In: Chapman C R, Loeser J D (eds) Issues in pain measurement. Raven Press, New York

Council J R, Ahern D K, Follick M J, Kline C L 1988 Expectancies and functional impairment in chronic low back pain. Pain 33: 323–331

Fairbank J C T, Couper J, Davies J B, O'Brien J P 1980 The Oswestry low back pain disability questionnaire. Physiotherapy 66: 271–273

Florey L L, Michelman S M 1982 Occupational role history: a screening tool for psychiatric occupational therapy. American Journal of Occupational Therapy 36: 301–308

Follick M J, Ahern D K, Laser-Wolston N 1984 Evaluation of a daily activity diary for chronic pain patients. Pain 19: 373–382

Fordyce W E, Lansky D, Calsyn D A, Shelton J L, Stolov W C, Rock D L 1984 Pain measurement and pain behaviour. Pain 18: 53–69

Gage M, Noh S, Polatajko H J, Kaspar V 1994 Measuring perceived self-efficacy in occupational therapy. American Journal of Occupational Therapy 48: 783–790

Grabois M, Blacker H M 1987 Chronic pain: measurement and assessment. International Journal of Rehabilitation 10: 265–270

Hemphill B J (ed) 1988 Mental health assessment in occupational therapy: an integrative approach to the evaluation process. Slack, Thoroughfare

Herda C A, Siegeris K, Basler H-D 1994 The pain beliefs and perceptions inventory: further evidence for a 4-factor structure. Pain 57: 85–90

Jensen M P, Karoly P 1987 Notes on the survey of pain attitudes (SOPA): original (24-item) and revised (35-item) versions. Unpublished manuscript. Arizona State University, Tempe

Jensen M P, Karoly P, Braver S 1986 The measurement of clinical pain intensity: a comparison of six methods. Pain 27: 117–126

Jensen M P, Karoly P, Huger R 1987 The development and preliminary validation of an instrument to assess patients' attitudes towards pain. Journal of Psychosomatic Research 31: 393–400

Johnstone M V, Keith R A, Hinderer S R 1992 Measurement standards for interdisciplinary medical rehabilitation. Archives of Physical Medicine and Rehabilitation 73: S3–S23

Karoly P 1985 The assessment of pain: concepts and procedures. In: Karoly P (ed) Measurement strategies in health psychology

Karoly P, Jensen M P 1987 Multimethod assessment of chronic pain. Pergamon Press, Oxford

Keefe F J 1987 Clinical pain assessment: implications for management. In: IASP refresher course on pain management. IASP, Hamburg

Keefe F J, Dolan E 1986 Pain behaviour and pain coping strategies in low back pain and myofacial pain dysfunction syndrome patients. Pain 24: 49–56

Kerns R D, Haythornthwaite J A 1988 Depression among chronic pain patients: cognitive-behavioural analysis and effect on rehabilitation outcome. Journal of Consulting and Clinical Psychology 56: 870–876

Kerns R D, Turk D C, Rudy T E 1985 The West Haven–Yale multidimensional pain inventory (WHYMPI). Pain 23: 345–356

Kielhofner G, Henry A 1988a The use of an occupational history interview in occupational therapy. In: Hemphill B J (ed) Mental health assessment in occupational therapy: an integrative approach to the evaluation process. Slack, Thoroughfare

Kielhofner G, Henry A 1988b Development and investigation of the occupational performance history interview. American Journal of Occupational Therapy 42: 489–498

Kielhofner G, Harlan B, Bauer D, Maurer P 1986 The reliability of a historical interview with physically disabled respondents. American Journal of Occupational Therapy 40: 551–556

Larrington G 1970 An exploratory study of the temporal aspects of adaptive functioning. Unpublished master's thesis, University of Southern California

Lindeman R H, Merenda P F 1979 Educational measurement, 2nd edn. Scott Foresman & Co, Glenview, Illinois

Lynch K B, Bridle M J 1993 Construct validity of the occupational performance history interview. Occupational Therapy Journal of Research 13: 231–240

McGrath P J, Unruh A M 1987 Pain in children and adolescents. Elsevier, Amsterdam

Main C J 1983 The modified somatic perception questionnaire (MSPQ). Journal of Psychosomatic Research 27: 503–514

Main C J, Waddell 1987 Psychometric construction and validity of the Pilowsky illness behaviour questionnaire in British patients with chronic low back pain. Pain 28: 13–25

Matsutsuyu J 1969 The interest checklist. American Journal of Occupational Therapy 23: 368–373

Melzack R 1975 The McGill pain questionnaire: major properties and scoring methods. Pain 1: 277–299

Melzack R, Torgerson W S 1971 On the language of pain. Anaesthiology 34: 50–59

Moore R 1990 Ethnographic assessment of pain coping perceptions. Psychomatic Medicine 52: 171–181

Moorehead L 1969 The occupational history. American Journal of Occupational Therapy 23: 329–338

Morley S, Wilkinson L 1995 The pain beliefs and perceptions inventory: a British replication. Pain 61: 427–433

National Health and Medical Research Council 1988 Management of severe pain. Australian Government Publishing Service, Canberra

Nicholas M 1994 Pain self-efficacy questionnaire (PSEQ): preliminary report. Unpublished paper, University of Sydney Pain Management and Research Centre, St Leonards

Pollard C A 1985 Preliminary validity study of the pain disability index. Perceptual and Motor Skills 59: 974

Pilowsky I, Spence N D 1983 Manual for the illness behaviour questionnaire (IBQ), 2nd edn. Department of Psychiatry, University of Adelaide

Rogers J 1988 The NPI interest checklist. In: Hemphill B J (ed) Mental health assessment in occupational therapy: an integrative approach to the evaluation process. Slack, Thoroughfare

Rosenstiel A K, Keefe F J 1983 The use of coping strategies in chronic low back pain patients: relationship to patient characteristics and current adjustment. Pain 17: 33–44

Rudy T E, Turk D C, Brena S F, Stieg R L, Brody M C 1990 Quantification of biomedical findings of chronic pain patients. Development of an index of pathology. Pain 42: 167–182

Sanders S H 1983 Automated versus self-monitoring of 'uptime' in chronic pain patients: a comparative study. Pain 15: 399–405

Scott J, Huskisson E C 1979 Vertical or horizontal visual analogue scale. Annals of the Rheumatic Diseases 38: 560

Strong J 1992a Chronic low back pain: towards an integrated psychosocial assessment. Unpublished PhD thesis, Department of Psychology, University of Queensland

Strong J 1992b Treatment strategies for patients with chronic low back pain. New Zealand Journal of Occupational Therapy 43: 3–6

Strong J 1995 Self-efficacy and patients with chronic low back pain. Moving in on Pain Conference, April, Adelaide

Strong J, Ashton R, Chant D 1991 Pain intensity measurement in chronic low back pain. Clinical Journal of Pain 7: 209–218

Strong J, Ashton R, Chant D 1992 The measurement of attitudes towards and beliefs about pain. Pain 48: 227–236

Strong J, Ashton R, Chant D, Cramond T 1994a Dimensions of chronic low back pain: the patients' perspectives. British Journal of Occupational Therapy 57: 204–208

Strong J, Ashton R, Stewart A 1994b Chronic low back pain: an integrated psychosocial assessment model. Journal of Counselling and Clinical Psychology 62: 1058–1063

Strong J, Large R G, Ashton R, Stewart A 1995 International replication study of the integrated psychosocial assessment model for patients with chronic low back pain. Clinical Journal of Pain 11: 296–306

Tait R C, Pollard C A, Margolis R B, Duckro P N, Krause S J 1987 The pain disability index: psychometric and validity data. Archives of Physical Medicine and Rehabilitation 68: 438–441

Tait R C, Chibnall J T, Krause S J 1990 The pain disability index: psychometric properties. Pain 40: 171–182

Turk D C, Kerns R D 1983 Conceptual issues in the assessment of clinical pain. International Journal of Psychiatry in Medicine 13: 57–68

Turk D C, Melzack R (eds) 1992 Handbook of pain assessment. Guilford, New York

Turk D C, Rudy T E 1987 Towards a comprehensive assessment of chronic pain patients. Behavioural Research Therapy 25: 237–249

Turk D C, Rudy T E 1988 Toward an empirically derived taxonomy of chronic pain patients: integration of psychological assessment data. Journal of Consulting and Clinical Psychology 56: 233–238

Vlaeyen J S, Snijders A M J, Schuerman J A, van Eck H, Groenman N H, Bremer J J C B 1989 Chronic pain and the three-systems model of emotions: a critical examination. Physical and Rehabilitation Medicine 1: 67–75

Waddell G 1987 Clinical assessment of lumbar impairment. Clinical Orthopaedics and Related Research 221: 110–120

Waddell G, Main C J 1984 Assessment of severity in low-back disorders. Spine 9: 204–208

Waddell G, Bircher M, Finlayson D, Main C J 1984a Symptoms and signs: physical disease or illness behaviour? British Medical Journal 289: 739–741

Waddell G, Main C J, Morris E W, Di Paola M, Gray I C M 1984b Chronic low-back pain, psychologic distress and illness behaviour. Spine 9: 209–213

Williams D A, Thorn B E 1989 An empirical assessment of pain beliefs. Pain 36: 351–358

Williams D A, Robinson M E, Geisser M E 1994 Pain beliefs: assessment and utility. Pain 59: 71–78

6

Scope of occupational therapy treatment

Function and the patient with pain 93
  Measuring function 93
  Methods 94
  Types of dysfunction 97
Work and the patient with pain 99
  Work, health and pain 101
  Occupational therapy and work – a
    brief history 102

Occupational therapy practice in the
  vocational arena 103
Efficacy of work rehabilitation and pain
  patients 107
Leisure and the patient with pain 109
Chapter summary 111
References 112

In this chapter, the impact which chronic pain can have upon the individual is considered in terms of well-known performance dimensions: activities of daily living (function), work, and leisure. The specific occupational therapy involvement in each of these performance areas is outlined and illustrated using pertinent case examples.

FUNCTION AND THE PATIENT WITH PAIN

This section considers ways of gauging the functional status of individuals with chronic pain, and the types of functional problems frequently experienced. The occupational therapy role in assisting clients to overcome functional disabilities is illustrated using a case example (see Box 6.1, p. 100).

Measuring function

Fisher (1992) has described function as referring '... primarily to the ability of the individual to perform the daily life tasks that he or she wants and needs to perform ...'. Some rehabilitation professionals are concerned with the client or patient's functional performance (Dunne 1993, Fisher 1992), while others may be more directed towards capability rather than performance – in the words of Verbrugge (1990), 'intrinsic rather than actual ability to do tasks'. A functional assessment may tap the relevant domains of personal activities of daily living (PADLs), instrumental activities of daily living (IADLs), work, rest and play. Usually though, measurement of function is confined to PADLs, some IADLs, and work abilities.

Methods

There are a number of ways to measure the functioning of the patient with chronic pain.

Questions

We may ask the patient to tell us about her activities. We frequently ask patients: 'Tell me what you did on a typical day prior to coming into hospital? What did you need to do, and what were you able to do? What did you have trouble doing? The answers give us some idea of the environmental demands placed upon the individual and the extent of their social disability. Social ability and disability relate to how the individual manages to perform personal and instrumental activities of daily living, work and leisure tasks (Verbrugge 1990).

Questionnaires

We may ask the patient to fill out an activities of daily living checklist. Either we ask the patient questions, using such measures as the Chronic Disability Index (Waddell & Main 1984), or we give them the questionnaire to complete. There is a multitude of scales available for such a purpose. There are also, nowadays, numerous self-report measures of functional ability allowing functional status measurement of pain patients (Deyo 1988, Hsieh et al 1992). They include the:

- Pain Disability Index (Pollard 1985, Tait et al 1987, 1990)
- Oswestry Low Back Pain Disability Index (Fairbank et al 1980)
- Chronic Disability Index (Waddell & Main 1984)
- Sickness Impact Profile (Bergner et al 1976, 1981)
- Functional Assessment Screening Questionnaire (Millard 1989).

There are, however, few data currently available to recommend the use of one functional status measure over the others (Deyo 1988), and there is certainly no single widely accepted, definitive disability measurement tool for use with patients (Watt-Watson & Graydon 1989).

Pain disability index. Two frequently used scales will be described here. The Pain Disability Index (PDI) is a self-report inventory which asks patients to rate on a scale from 0 to 10 the degree to which pain interferes with functioning in seven areas of daily living (Pollard 1985, Tait et al 1987, 1990). Apart from the 1985 report which used 18 patients with low back pain, the other two studies on the PDI have used patients with heterogeneous pain complaints. More recently, the PDI has been examined for use both with patients with heterogeneous pain complaints (Jerome & Gross 1991) and with patients with chronic low back pain (Gronblad et al 1993). It is a frequently used research measure (see, for example, the study by Peters & Large 1990).

Oswestry low back pain disability questionnaire (OLBPDQ). The Oswestry Low Back Pain Disability Questionnaire (OLBPDQ) consists of nine functional categories and a pain intensity scale (Fairbank et al 1980). Each category is scored on a 0–5 scale, where 5 represents the greatest disability. Thus far, only a cursory examination has been made of the psychometric properties of the OLBPDQ. As noted by McDowell and Newell (1987) when reviewing the OLBPDQ: 'The preliminary nature of the validity and reliability tests, however, indicates that further analyses need to be carried out to assess the quality of this measurement'. No Cronbach's coefficients have been reported; nor has an examination been made of its underlying factor structure. Its content validity has not been demonstrated (DeLitto 1989). Yet it remains widely used (see, for example, the study by Hurri 1989). Other work examining this scale has used a modified Oswestry *and not the original questionnaire* (see, for example Baker et al 1989, Hudson-Cook et al 1989).

PDI and OLBPDQ comparisons. Gronblad and his colleagues (1993) examined the comparability of the Pain Disability Index and the Oswestry Low Back Pain Disability Questionnaire in terms of scale intercorrelations and test–retest reliability.

We (Strong et al 1994) also undertook a comparative examination of the reliability and validity of these two frequently used self-report measures of functional disability. We used a descriptive ex-post facto design. 100 patients with chronic low back pain of non-cancer origin were administered the two questionnaires as part of a larger questionnaire battery. Acceptable internal consistency values of 0.76 for the PDI and 0.71 for the OLBPDQ were obtained. A correlation of $r = 0.63$ was found between the PDI and the OLBPDQ, supporting the concurrent validity of the two scales. Both scales were found to be correlated to the Beck Depression Inventory scores (for PDI, $r = 0.42$, and for OLBPDQ, $r = 0.39$), with higher disability associated with greater depression. Only the total PDI score was found to be sensitive to functional status differences within the patient sample. Findings of the study add support to other recent work in favour of the PDI.

More recently, Gronblad and his colleagues (1994) compared the relationship between a patient's perceived disability on the PDI and the OLBPDQ and actual performance on tests of physical function. They found a significant relationship, with more support being given to the PDI.

The use of self-report measures of functional ability and disability is a standard part of practice with patients with chronic pain. As was established in Chapter 5, with any rehabilitation practice area, it is necessary for such measures to be reliable and valid (Johnstone et al 1992). Taken together, the studies we have reviewed here provide good support for the reliability and sensitivity of the Pain Disability Index as a self-report measure of functional status in the patient with chronic pain.

Disability and depression. An interesting consideration here is the relationship between perceived disability and dysfunction and depression (Strong et al 1994). In our study, the function scales were highly positively correlated with depression. The more depressed the patients were, the more disability was perceived. This relationship is an important one, of which occupational therapists should be aware. Turk and his colleagues (1987) discussed the possible overlap between symptoms of depression and symptoms of chronic medical conditions such as chronic pain. Alternatively, it could be that, when depressed, individual patients tended to answer a self-report questionnaire such as the PDI through the cognitively distorted view of themselves as being helpless and hopeless. Certainly, such a relationship warrants closer attention.

Observation of function

We may ask the patient to perform some functional task, and observe their performance. For example, we may ask the patient to complete an obstacle course, to engage in a group activity, to complete a speed walk, or to prepare a meal, and observe their functioning. This will give us an idea of their physical and social disability.

Activity diary

We may ask the patient to keep an activity diary, in which they record what they do every half hour or hour (Fordyce 1976). Often, patients are asked to keep an activity diary in the weeks prior to admission to a pain management program. This gives us a measure of social disability.

Covert observation

We may ask ward staff to unobtrusively observe the patient every hour and make a regular record of the patient's activity level (Kremer et al 1981).

Automated measures

We may use some automated measure of a patient's activity levels. Original work in this area relied on stationary devices attached to beds or chairs to automatically record downtime (Cairns et al 1976). (Downtime refers to the amount of time the patient spends lying or sitting, while its corollary, uptime, is the amount of time the patient spends walking or standing (Sanders 1980).) Sanders (1980, 1983) reported on the development of an uptime device for chronic pain patients. Further work on uptime has been conducted by Follick and his colleagues (1985) and White and Strong (1992).

Assessment of physical parameters

We may assess physical performance parameters such as range of motion (Verbrugge 1990). Harding and her colleagues (1994) reported on the development of a battery of measures which can be used to assess the physical function of patients with chronic pain. Their method involves direct sampling of an individual's behaviour under controlled conditions. After examining the reliability and validity of a number of measures of physical function, Harding et al (1994) recommended a 30-minute procedure which includes distance walking for 5 minutes, stair climbing for 1 minute, getting in and out of a chair for 1 minute, and an endurance measure for holding the arms in the horizontal plane.

Assessment of work abilities

We may assess the patient's work abilities, and residual functional capacities (Abdel-Moty et al 1993, Callaghan 1993). This will be dealt with in more detail in the work section of this chapter (p. 101).

Types of dysfunction

A reduction in the functional activity of the individual is a frequent consequence of chronic pain. Occupational therapists can use the results from a measure such as the Pain Disability Index to guide further enquiry and intervention. Areas where dysfunction occurs include self-care activities, sexual activities and instrumental activities. Greater difficulties are usually to be found with instrumental than with personal activities of daily living. (This is not to suggest that no individual with chronic pain has difficulty with personal activities of daily living.)

When working with dysfunction, I have found Verbrugge's (1990) definition of disability – 'the gap between a person's capability and the environment's demand' – to be particularly helpful. Implicit in this definition is the possibility of intervention on both sides of the equation, that is, interventions to modify the individual's capacity, or interventions to modify the demands of the environment. The occupational therapist can help in both of these areas, by improving the person's capabilities or by modifying the task or environment.

Self-care

If a patient indicates that she has difficulty with self-care tasks, further enquiry may reveal that the patient (in this case, a woman with right upper limb reflex sympathetic dystrophy) has difficulty with some dressing tasks (bra and stockings), because moving her right arm is exquisitely painful. As her occupational therapist, you may initially try to help her to use her right arm more by, for example, a combination of relaxation, gravity eliminated movements and bilateral activities. (Concurrent with your intervention, the patient would typically be seen by a physiotherapist and an anaesthetist.) If the strategy to increase functional pain-free movement of her arm is unsuccessful, then you would suggest modifications to the tasks (one-handed dressing techniques). Such a sequential approach is preferred, since the primary goal is to encourage normal movements of her affected arm, thereby minimizing problems of disuse. If, however, such an approach fails, then the second goal of therapy is to increase function by alternative techniques.

Sexual activity

Sexual activity has been classed by some as a personal activity of daily living and by others as an instrumental activity of daily living. Kennedy (1987) has preferred to include sexual activity within the performance area of leisure or recreation. Whatever its classification, sexual activity is an activity which many individuals with chronic pain find difficult. Buckwalter and her colleagues (1982) observed that 'Many patients with musculoskeletal disorders are hindered in their sexual expression' – one only needs to remember the old adage 'Not tonight dear, I have a headache' to realize that head pain and sexual activity do not sit well together. So it is with many other types of pain, including back pain, neck pain, upper limb pain and abdominal pain.

Most attention to the existence of sexual problems has been given to those individuals with back pain. Labbe (1988) observed that patients with back pain may have unique sexual problems. Sjögren and Fugl-Meyer (1981) found an increase in sexual dysfunction in men and women after the onset of chronic back pain. Patients with chronic back pain may have sexual problems due to both direct and indirect effects (Ritchie & Daines 1992). Direct effects may be due to difficulties maintaining particular positions, an inability to support the partner's weight or difficulty performing the movement associated with intercourse (Ritchie & Daines 1992). Indirect effects may be due to fear of further pain or injury, loss of self-esteem, loss of libido, or the effects of depression and/or medication (Ritchie & Daines 1992). An additional complication can be the strain put upon relationships, and the concern that partners will go outside the relationship for gratification. For people in pain who are not already in relationships, the concerns can be equally great.

Kennedy (1987) suggests that occupational therapists utilize a rehabilitative frame of reference when helping clients to adjust to sexual changes after physical disability. With the aid of a back pain leaflet which describes positions of comfort for intercourse, and the use of supportive cushions and pillows, occupational therapists are able to assist patients with simple sexual counselling (Ritchie & Daines 1992). The *Back to Sex* package (1985) is another resource which can be used with patients with back pain. Similar assistance using rehabilitative techniques such as work simplification, joint protection, task adaptation and environmental adaptation (Kennedy 1987), can be given to patients with other types of chronic pain who are experiencing sexual dysfunction.

Instrumental activity

Instrumental activities cover a wide variety of activities such as home maintenance, mobility within the environment, interacting with others, budgeting and shopping. Individuals with chronic pain may experience difficulties in many areas. If we think once again of our female patient with right upper limb reflex sympathetic dystrophy, she may have difficulty with meal preparation, changing the baby's nappy, house cleaning, hanging up the washing, ironing, driving the manual car, and getting the groceries.

Occupational therapy intervention in the area of instrumental activities can include increasing the patient's activity tolerance, performing instrumental activities though a graded activity program, education in work simplification techniques and good body mechanics, so the patient can complete tasks (for example, meal preparation) with greater ease, and the provision of adaptive equipment (for example, long-handled dustpans and brushes), so that essential tasks can be performed without bending. The patient may also benefit from:

- Assistance with time management – how to structure the day/week.
- Assertiveness training, to enable the patient to get appropriate help from family members.
- Assistance with problem solving; for example, how to get help with parcel and grocery deliveries.

The case example in Box 6.1 illustrates the occupational therapy role in assisting clients to overcome functional disability.

WORK AND THE PATIENT WITH PAIN

Occupational therapists provide preventive, evaluative, remediative, restorative and compensatory services that are designed to improve the functional work status of individuals in all age groups (American Occupational Therapy Association 1992).

Work is fundamental to occupational therapy thinking and is considered to be of crucial importance by occupational therapists, partly because of the contribution it makes to role identity. How many times in our daily lives

> **Box 6.1** The case of Ms J
>
> Ms J was a 35-year-old woman who, at the time of presentation for occupational therapy, was living with her parents. She had had chronic low back pain and left-sided sciatica for 8 years since being injured in a motor vehicle accident. She was diagnosed as having arachnoiditis. Her occupation was a university student, although at the time of presentation for occupational therapy she had deferred her studies.
>
> *Assessment*
> Assessment on the Pain Disability Index revealed the following:
> - life-support activities: 3/10, with difficulty sleeping and getting out of bed
> - self-care activities: 8/10, with problems with showering, dressing, and walking
> - sexual activities: not applicable
> - social activities: 8/10, with difficulties sitting in the car to visit friends
> - family/home responsibilities: 2/10, with minimal problems seen here since her parents had assumed most tasks
> - recreation: 8/10, only able to listen to music and read, but holding books was a problem
> - work: 9/10, with problems with getting to classes, holding books, sitting in lectures, doing assignments.
>
> An overall disability score of 38/70 was obtained.
>
> *Intervention*
> Occupational therapy intervention with Ms J was focused on modifying her tasks and the environment in the following ways:
> *Bedroom.* Assessment was made for a supportive bed, the room was rearranged and a sturdy dressing-table was placed next to the bed, so that Ms J could pull herself up off the bed. She was shown how to roll onto her side and swing her legs over the side of the bed to help her get out of bed.
> *Bathroom.* Information was given on the use of a long-handled sponge, soap-on-rope, non-slip surface and grab rail for shower. It was suggested that Ms J should sit to perform lower limb dressing, using a dressing stick.
> *Study.* It was recommended that Ms J use a bookrest for reading, information was given about an architect's bench, and her computer area was rearranged to ensure good workbench heights. An office chair with good back support and five star base was recommended.
> *Car.* The use of a back support was recommended, and Ms J was taught an easier method to get into and out of her car.
> These recommendations were followed by Ms J with the outcome that she became more independent and comfortable in performing relevant activities of daily living. She did not return to her university studies.

have we heard conversations that begin 'So what do you do?' or, 'Where do you work?' As Kielhofner said: 'When an activity is considered to be one's work, it is generally organised into a major life role' (1983, cited in Cromwell 1985–1986). In this section, we first examine the relationships between work, health and pain. A brief historical sketch of occupational therapy involvement in work is then drawn. Areas of occupational therapy involvement in the work arena for people with pain problems are considered, and highlighted using case examples. Finally, we examine the efficacy of work programs for individuals with chronic pain.

Work, health and pain

'Work is an essential part of life' (MacDonald 1976). It provides individuals with economic, psychological, physical and social benefits (Anthony & Blanch 1987). Economic benefits may include money and future income security (such as pensions or superannuation). Psychological benefits derived from work include self-esteem, satisfaction, participation, belonging and challenge. Physical benefits can include activity and exercise. Social benefits include social contacts and involvement.

What then of work and the patient with chronic pain? We have established earlier that individuals with chronic pain frequently experience a reduction in their levels of functioning. Work is one of the areas of functioning which is almost invariably disrupted. As Richardson et al (1994) note: 'Loss of paid work or other vocational activity is a common accompaniment of chronic pain'. Lehmann et al (1993) found that 16% of their sample of 55 patients with acute low back pain had not returned to work at a 6-month follow-up. Strong (1992) found that only 7% of a sample of 100 patients with chronic low back pain remained in the paid workforce.

Feuerstein (1991) has presented a model of work disability for occupational musculoskeletal injuries which highlights the interaction between a patient's disorder, her physical capabilities, the ergonomic demands and psychosocial variables (see Fig. 6.1). All such factors can influence outcome after an occupational injury. Such a model has much to offer in the rehabilitation of individuals with chronic pain. We will return to this model in a later section (p. 103).

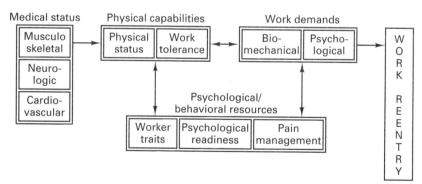

Figure 6.1 A model of work disability for occupational musculoskeletal injuries, illustrating the factors that can affect return to work. (Adapted from Feuerstein 1991, with permission.)

Occupational therapy and work – a brief history

Occupational therapy as a profession was founded on a belief in the importance of occupation for the health of individuals. Polatajko (1992) spoke eloquently of this in the 1992 Muriel Driver Lecture. Using the poignant case example of an individual denied occupation through severe Guillain–Barré disease, Polatajko showed how the woman's inability to 'do' was intrinsically linked to her will to live or not live.

Over the years, work has been, and remains, an important evaluative tool and therapeutic medium for the occupational therapist (Ogden & Wright 1985). While occupational therapists such as Kielhofner (1983) have used 'work' as a broad term which can encompass all productive activities, not just those which are reimbursed, in this section the term is used to refer to vocational or paid activities.

A number of authors have provided a detailed historical account of occupational therapy involvement in work (see, for example, Cromwell 1985–1986, Hanson & Walker 1992, Ogden & Wright 1985). In this section, the key points of occupational therapy involvement with work will be made. However, for a comprehensive coverage, the reader is directed to the references cited.

Occupational therapy had its beginnings in the 'Moral Treatment' era of the late 19th century (Cromwell 1985–1986), which emphasized the engagement of patients with mental illness in manual work, recreation and self-care (Cromwell 1985–1986, Hanson & Walker 1992). With the advent of World War I, the demand for occupational therapists to assist in the rehabilitation of injured soldiers fostered the development of the profession (Anderson & Bell 1988, Canadian Association of Occupational Therapists 1988, Hanson & Walker 1992, Ogden & Wright 1985).

In the United States of America in 1920, the Vocational Rehabilitation Act came into force (Cromwell 1985–1986, Hanson & Walker 1992); it aimed to return patients to paid employment, and became the cornerstone of the development of vocational rehabilitation services in America (Hanson & Walker 1992).

With the arrival of World War II, occupational therapy was again given a boost, with demand for the rehabilitation of injured service personnel. Anderson and Bell (1988) observed that occupational therapy as an Australian profession was born at this time.

After the war, many occupational therapists abandoned their focus on work in favour of more medically oriented interventions (Hanson & Walker 1992), psychoanalytically oriented interventions (Cromwell 1985–1986), or 'devicing' treatments (Cromwell 1985–1986). It was not until the late 1970s that occupational therapists again directed their attention to the importance of work and vocational rehabilitation for patients with injuries or disabilities (Hanson & Walker 1992).

Occupational therapists bring to the vocational rehabilitation area their knowledge of clinical conditions, their skills of task analysis and their understanding of role demands on the individual (Canadian Association of Occupational Therapists 1988). Our background knowledge of physical and psychosocial rehabilitation is invaluable in vocational rehabilitation (Smith et al 1986). Ogden and Wright (1985) identified a number of reasons for the involvement of occupational therapists in the work-related rehabilitation of patients with industrial injuries, including:

1. The underlying occupational therapy philosophy advocates the use of work as a therapeutic medium.
2. Occupational therapists, with an undergraduate training in biomedical and psychosocial aspects of health, are ideally prepared to do work evaluation and work hardening.
3. The ability to return to work needs more than traditional rehabilitation.
4. The prediction of ability to return to work needs more than psychometric testing.
5. Evaluating a client using 'real' work activities will yield details about not only the worker's physical capabilities but also her work habits. (Ogden & Wright 1985).

Occupational therapy practice in the vocational arena

Occupational therapy literature documents the following occupational therapy services in the vocational arena (Hook 1985–1986):

- functional capacity evaluation
- work capacity evaluation
- work tolerance screening
- work hardening
- job analysis
- on-the-job assessment
- job site modification or worker modification
- job search skills training
- corporate consultation.

Each of these services addresses the various facets of Feuerstein's (1991) model for return to work. These areas will now be considered, and illustrated with case examples. It must be noted that the case examples have been provided to illustrate a particular service. In reality, the total occupational therapy program would not usually have considered one technique in isolation.

Functional capacity evaluation (FCE)

Some confusion exists in the literature about what is encompassed by the term 'functional capacity evaluation' (Gibson 1994). Velozo (1993) has suggested that the term covers both physical capacity evaluation and work capacity evaluation. In her comprehensive review of FCE, Gibson (1994) defined it as the process of measuring a person's capacity for sustained performance of broadly defined physical work demands.

Work capacity evaluation (WCE)

A work capacity evaluation is the measurement of a person's 'capacity to dependably sustain [work] demands' (Holmes 1985). WCE involves a client in an intensive, individualized assessment program, the length of which may vary. For example, Hook (1985–1986) reported a program with 6-hour days for a minimum of 5 days up to a maximum of 10 days. Meanwhile, Ogden and Wright (1985) reported a 2-week program for WCE. During a WCE, clients perform various activities under supervision. Velozo (1993) has suggested that the work capacity evaluation is more comprehensive than a physical capacity evaluation in that an assessment is made of performance requiring several functional units (for example, lifting as opposed to grasp). A WCE goes further than looking at the worker's performance at the functional unit level. It also looks at the worker's interests, aptitudes, work tolerances, fatigue tolerance, flexibility, muscle endurance, temperament, attitudes and work skills (Holmes 1985, Hook 1985–1986). Thus, a WCE yields information about the client's physical work tolerances, and her worker characteristics and feasibility (Ogden & Wright 1985). Work tasks considered may include lifting, standing, sitting, walking, pushing, pulling and carrying (Velozo 1993).

WCE typically makes use of criterion-referenced tests, which give information on a person's ability to perform a particular activity (Jacobs 1991). This is in comparison to a norm-referenced test, which considers the individual subject's performance compared to a standardized sample (Jacobs 1991). Evaluation may be made using specific equipment such as Valpar, WEST (Ogden-Niemeyer 1991).

Work tolerance screening (WTS)

Work tolerance screening has been described as 'a physical and functional assessment of the injured worker' (Holmes 1985). In many settings, WTS is used as the initial evaluation for all clients referred to the centre (Ogden & Wright 1985).

Characteristics of WTS include a short but intensive evaluation, the time frame of which may be 1 hour to 1 day (Holmes 1985), 3–4 hours

> **Box 6.2** Case example of WTS
>
> A 29-year-old woman with a low back injury was referred for WTS. The client had injured her back 1 year previously while working as a part-time cook. A 3-hour WTS evaluation was undertaken by the occupational therapist. This evaluation included a review of medical history and symptoms, an examination of the client's use of time, and an assessment of neurological and muscular functioning. An assessment of the client's ability to use small hand tools at various heights and lift weighted objects at various heights was then performed. Results of this WTS supported a gradual return to work plan for the client (DeRenne-Stephan 1985).

(Ogden & Wright 1985), or 3–7 hours per day for 3 weeks (Hook 1985–1986). During a WTS, a client's performance on a number of critical physical demands is measured (Holmes 1985, Ogden & Wright 1985). These are the demands of the job thought most likely to produce symptoms which will limit a worker's tolerance.

The evaluation will consider the worker's range of motion, muscle strength, grip strength, dexterity, sensory status, tolerance to temperature and vibration, ability to lift and carry under load, and ability to apply torque with different tools (Hook 1985–1986). The results of a WTS will provide useful baseline information about a client's specific abilities and tolerances (Holmes 1985, Hook 1985–1986).

A case example from DeRenne-Stephan (1985) is given in Box 6.2.

Work hardening (WH)

The American Occupational Therapy Association (1986) described work hardening as 'a work-oriented treatment program designed to improve the client's productivity'. The interested reader is referred to a number of excellent texts in the area of work hardening (see, for example, American Occupational Therapy Association 1986, Ogden-Niemeyer & Jacobs 1989).

While the term 'work hardening' was coined during the 1980s, this activity has parallels in the progressive grading of activities used by therapists for patients with physical disabilities in the clinical setting (Holmes 1985). Occupational therapy training and experience provides a suitable background for this area of practice (King 1992). By using WH techniques, occupational therapists can help to match the client's functional capacity with the specific demands of the job (Wyrick et al 1991).

Work hardening programs utilize real or simulated work activities in addition to activities designed to improve biomechanical, cardiovascular, psychosocial, and neuromuscular functioning (Wyrick et al 1991). Hook (1985–1986) has described a work hardening program where clients participated for 3 weeks (commencing with 2 hours per day and building

> **Box 6.3** Case example of WH
>
> A client with low back pain was participating in a work hardening program. The 32-year-old client had a 16-month history of low back pain, combined with right knee pain and swelling. Occupational therapy WH goals for the client were to increase sitting, standing, lifting and lowering tolerances, and to increase the client's knowledge of good body mechanics.

up to 6 hours per day). Work hardening aims to increase worker productivity by decreasing secondary impairments, functional limitations, disability and vocational handicap, while at the same time improving vocational feasibility and employability (Matheson et al 1985).

King (1992) has pointed out that the area of work hardening has become increasingly specialized. After conducting a survey of 242 American occupational therapists employed in work hardening programs, she suggested that educational programs for occupational therapists should incorporate more up-to-date training on work hardening.

A recent paper in The American Journal of Occupational Therapy (Callaghan 1993) presented the case report given in Box 6.3.

Job analysis (JA)

Job analysis is a detailed evaluation made of the physical, environmental and psychosocial demands of a specific job (Hook 1985–1986, Ogden & Wright 1985). An examination is made of the employment setting in which the client works and the operational characteristics of the job (Hook 1985–1986). It has been my experience and that of others (see Hook 1985–1986, for example) that a job analysis by the occupational therapist can reveal hitherto unobserved factors which may impact upon a person's performance (as in the case example given in Box 6.4).

> **Box 6.4** Case example of JA
>
> Mrs D was employed as a secretary when she experienced upper limb, neck and head pains. A provisional diagnosis of occupational overuse was noted. Job analysis was undertaken by the occupational therapist.
>
> Mrs D had a varied work routine. There were times in the week when the workload was greatly increased. At these times, Mrs D became very stressed. On most occasions, she was the sole occupant of the office. Duties performed included typing correspondence and memos on an electric typewriter, answering the telephone, dealing with queries from the public, making appointments, and typing reports onto the word processor. Mrs D was right hand dominant and wore bifocal glasses.
>
> The layout of the office provided two main work areas – a general desk with an electric typewriter at one side, and another desk with a word processor. Being an internal room, the office was lit by artificial lighting, and ventilated by desk fans.

> **Box 6.4** cont'd
>
> When sitting at either the general desk or the computer desk, Mrs D sat on a vinyl covered chair with a four-castor base. The seat height was 19.5 inches. A firm 3-inch cushion was placed on the chair. The height of the typewriter keys was 30.5 inches from floor level. The height of both desks was 26.5 inches. The VDU screen was currently elevated on two sets of 'telephone books' (5 inches). There was no document holder, and Mrs D had to turn her neck frequently to the right to read the manuscripts.
>
> Suggestions to assist Mrs D focused on the physical environment and the organizational environment. It was suggested that a VDU workstation, a document holder and a gas lift chair with a five-castor base should be purchased. In terms of organizational change, methods to regulate the flow of work into the office were explored. Prioritizing of work tasks and deadlines for work submission were established, and the possibility of getting in temporary assistance at peak periods was raised.

On-the-job assessment

An on-the-job (or worksite) assessment of the client may be made, in which the occupational therapist observes the client's endurance, pain tolerance and performance in the specific job setting (Hook 1985–1986). From such an assessment, necessary modifications to the job-site or the worker can be made (Hook 1985–1986). A case example is given in Box 6.5.

Efficacy of work rehabilitation and pain patients

As with all areas of occupational therapy intervention with patients with chronic pain conditions, we must ask 'How effective are these various aspects of work intervention?' We need to go beyond the anecdotal case report in order to look at the efficacy of such approaches. In this section, we will look briefly at the efficacy of work-related interventions with patients with pain problems, bearing in mind the difficulty in examining the efficacy of single components in isolation.

Niemeyer et al (1994) examined return-to-work rates of industrial rehabilitation programs over a 10-year period, and found figures ranging from 60–80% for program participants. However, after noting differences in study design, program acceptance criteria, client characteristics, type of injury, length of time off work, and type of outcome, this group developed an (American) National Work-Hardening Outcome Study, conducted by the American Occupational Therapy Association Special Interest Section Work Programs Group. 36 work hardening programs participated in an outcome survey using a sequential case series design. Each centre completed a survey on each of 10 consecutive referrals. Of the 220 clients who completed a work hardening program, 75.9% returned to work and

> **Box 6.5** Case example of worksite assessment
>
> Mr K was a 40-year-old man who was trained as a motor mechanic. 18 months previously, while working as a maintenance person, he had fallen onto his sacrum/coccyx. Opinions from specialists indicated Mr K had a pre-existing condition of lumbar spondylosis which had been aggravated by the fall. After treatment on a pain management program, he was entered on a work assessment scheme by the relevant workers compensation organization. It was at this time that a referral was received by the occupational therapist for a worksite assessment. Excerpts from the worksite assessment report follow:
>
> *Job title.* Mower mechanic
> *Job task.* Repairing broken mowers and renovating old mowers for resale
> *Job description.* Worker must walk 25 feet to room outside the workshop to collect a mower for repair. Worker returns to his bench inside the workshop pushing the mower in front of him. Mower must be lifted up from concrete floor onto 37.5-inch-high workbench. The worker is unable to lift a mower onto workbench unaided. After he obtains help to lift mower up, the worker stands at bench to inspect and work on mower. Mower parts are held in bench vice on workbench. Tools are located in wall cupboards or display boards mounted on wall above bench. Worker, who is 6 feet 4 inches tall, can easily reach tools he requires. Mower parts are located 10 feet away in cupboards. Worker can access these parts, in some cases needing to bend his knees to reach objects on lower shelves. Worker is unable to independently turn mower over to work on its underside on the workbench. At times, the worker sits on high stool at his workbench, while at other times he stands with a wide base gait, and at other times he rests one foot on a footstool. At completion of benchwork, worker needs assistance to lift mower back to floor.
>
> The physical demands of the job include walking short distances periodically, reaching tools at the back of 22-inch-wide benches, stooping to obtain some parts, working at bench for extended periods, pushing mowers on concrete floor, having good eye–hand coordination and bilateral upper limb dexterity, and lifting mowers from floor to bench, from bench to floor, and turning mowers over on bench.
>
> Mr K is able to cope adequately with all physical demands of the job except for the lifting of mowers. Since this is an integral part of the operation of a mower repair man, suggest the modification of the work-task by the purchase and use of a mower hoist to allow worker to independently lift, turn and lower mower.

24.1% did not return to work. These figures are encouraging. As expected, the longer the time off work, the poorer the outcome.

Tollison (1991) compared the outcome of a hospital-based occupational rehabilitation program for patients with occupational low back pain, with a non-treatment group. 44 patients treated in a 20-hour functional restoration program were compared with 20 people denied treatment by insurance companies. It was found that significantly more treated patients had returned to work at 12 months (59% of the treatment group vs 20% of the non-treated group).

Riipinen et al (1994) examined studies of vocational rehabilitation outcome for patients with musculoskeletal deficits reported between 1980 and 1990. 23 suitable studies were retrieved by a MedLine search, of which six could be classified as rehabilitation to alleviate chronic pain. From these studies, the percentage reporting a positive effect on work status ranged from 15–55%.

Gallagher et al (1989) examined the determinants of return to work among 150 subjects with chronic low back pain. A 6-month follow-up was conducted for 87 patients treated at a low back pain clinic and 63 people who had not yet received treatment. 41% of clinic patients as compared to 16% of non-clinic patients had returned to work at 6 months. Interestingly, Gallagher et al found that the results of the physical examination and biomechanical testing were not predictors of resultant employment status (when age and length of time off work were controlled). It was the psychosocial factors rather than the physical factors which had an impact on employment outcome. This finding reinforces the point I made earlier (Ch. 5), that a comprehensive assessment needs to be made of the person with chronic pain. To rely solely on a physical assessment is not advisable, as Gallagher and his colleagues illustrated.

LEISURE AND THE PATIENT WITH PAIN

While one person's leisure may be considered someone else's work, there are, nevertheless, some factors which can be attributed to leisure activities. Shaw (1985) has suggested that a leisure activity may contain the components of enjoyment, lack of evaluation, relaxation, freedom of choice and intrinsic motivation. Very little attention has been given in the literature to the topic of leisure/recreation and individuals with chronic pain. While the literature and actual practice do not follow an exact relationship, I suggest that the lack of attention to leisure in the pain literature has a parallel in practice. Leisure, when it is considered in clinical settings such as pain clinics, is often seen as a non-essential, if not frivolous, extra. Lyons (1987) observed that general rehabilitation programs for people with chronic illness or disability place a greater emphasis on physical functioning than on leisure functioning. In busy clinical settings, the focus upon essential functions like ADLs and work has the highest priority.

I would suggest that a number of factors point to the importance of paying attention to the leisure functioning of our patients with pain. Writers such as Coleman (1993) have suggested that leisure may act as a type of coping resource to help deal with life stressors (ongoing pain is seen to be a source of considerable stress for many patients with pain). In addition, many patients with chronic pain seen at pain clinics are no longer employed and have a great deal of time on their hands. Avocational pursuits may therefore comprise a large proportion of their daily activities.

In this section we draw on the available literature and clinical experience to describe some of the leisure deficits which individuals with chronic pain can experience, and to provide some guidelines to consider in practice.

For many individuals with a chronic illness or disability, a problem can arise with the increase in discretionary time. Let us consider the case example of Mr Y (Box 6.6).

The words of Sir Ludwig Guttman (1976) when describing leisure pursuit, are particularly pertinent to our consideration of leisure for persons with chronic pain: 'The great advantage of sport over formal remedial exercise lies in its recreational value, which represents an additional motivation for the disabled [person] by restoring that passion for playful activity and the desire to experience joy and pleasure in life, so deeply inherent in any human being'.

Individuals with chronic pain may find it difficult to engage in many physically oriented leisure pursuits. Vigorous movements can be problematic; twisting movements (such as are found, for example, in games like golf) can be difficult, and pounding movements (such as occur in jogging) can aggravate pain. Yet Sharpe et al (1988), in a review, noted that jogging has been advocated as protecting individuals with back pain by increasing the 'strength and endurance of the postural muscles'.

Even sedentary activities may be problematic for many individuals with chronic pain; activities which require sustained concentration (for example, playing chess) may be difficult, as may activities which need one to maintain a static position for a considerable length of time (for example, attending the theatre).

Box 6.6 The case of Mr Y

Mr Y, a 26-year-old man, had sustained a left brachial plexus lesion following a motor bike accident. Prior to his injury, Mr Y had been a motor bike enthusiast; his main recreational pursuits were associated with motor bikes – tinkering with his bike, restoring an old bike in his garage, riding his bike with his mates at weekends, and drinking with his mates. Since the injury 2 years ago, Mr Y had been unable to continue in his former job as a factory worker. He had been on sickness benefits, and had a dramatic increase in the amount of discretionary time available to him. However, he felt unable, due to the combined problem of a flail left arm and the attendant unrelenting pain, to engage in most of his previous leisure pursuits. As Lyons (1987) said, such discretionary time can be used productively and yield feelings of satisfaction, or it can be misused and result in boredom and negative feelings. In the case of Mr Y, the only remaining leisure interest he could identify was drinking with his mates, which he engaged in frequently. He also began drinking on his own, to fill the time and to give some relief from the pain. He was filled with feelings of despair, and just wanted to be rid of the pain. We will return to the case of Mr Y in Box 6.7.

There is no list prescribing which leisure pursuits are 'best' for the person with chronic pain. Rather, the occupational therapist is advised to ask the patient about her recreational activities – remember that this can be screened by one of the items on the Pain Disability Index which was described earlier (p. 94). An individual approach is recommended for each patient. Lyons (1987) has suggested that an examination should be made of the person's current leisure behaviour to determine the type of activities perceived as leisure, the degree and nature of their current involvement, and the location, time and social milieu in which such leisure takes place. A comparison between the individual's current and previous leisure engagement and satisfaction levels can then be made, and any desired changes to leisure behaviours can be determined, taking into consideration anything which may be a barrier to success (Lyons 1987).

Let us return to the case of Mr Y (Box 6.6, Box 6.7).

CHAPTER SUMMARY

In this chapter, we examined the ways in which chronic pain can interfere with an individual's competence in the performance areas of activities of daily living, work and leisure. These are, all of them, fundamental areas of occupational therapy concern. Given that, very often, individuals with chronic pain do experience difficulty in some, if not all performance areas, it is important for the occupational therapist to be well versed in these areas so that patients' performance skills may be enhanced as far as possible, and so that they are able to attain an improved quality of life. In Chapter 7, we examine particular techniques which the occupational therapist can use to help patients with pain achieve such increases in function.

Box 6.7 The case of Mr Y (continued)

Currently, Mr Y perceives a 9/10 recreation disability due to his pain (using the Pain Disability Index). The only one of his former leisure activities he now engages in is drinking with his mates. His interests lie with motor bikes and little else. The occupational therapist may work with Mr Y to analyse the types of tasks involved in tinkering with bikes, or bike restoration. She may advise environmental adaptations such as using a workbench at the correct height, so Mr Y can prop himself on a stool and tinker with the bike bits, using a tool such as a vice to stabilize parts while he works with his right hand (fortunately, he is right hand dominant). The occupational therapist can also help Mr Y to explore how he can use his interest in motor bikes in a different way – perhaps researching the history of his particular bike. Of course, while the occupational therapist is exploring leisure options with Mr Y, Mr Y would be undergoing a comprehensive multidisciplinary pain management program.

REFERENCES

Abdel-Moty E, Fishbain D A, Khalil T M, Sadek S, Cutler R, Rosomoff R S, Rosomoff H L 1993 Functional capacity and residual functional capacity and their utility in measuring work capacity. Clinical Journal of Pain 9: 168–173

American Occupational Therapy Association 1986 Work hardening guidelines. American Journal of Occupational Therapy 40: 841–843

American Occupational Therapy Association 1992 Statement: occupational therapy services in work practice. American Journal of Occupational Therapy 46: 1086–1088

Anderson B, Bell J 1988 Occupational therapy: its place in Australia's history. New South Wales Association of Occupational Therapists, Sydney

Anthony W A, Blanch A 1987 Supported employment for persons who are psychiatrically disabled: a historical and conceptual perspective. Psychosocial Rehabilitation Journal 11: 5–23

Back to sex: lower back pain and sexuality [videorecording] 1985 Medical Communications Unit, Royal Newcastle Hospital in association with the Hunter Region Rehabilitation services, Newcastle, NSW

Baker D J, Pynsent P B, Fairbank J C T 1987 The Oswestry disability index revisited: its reliability, repeatability and validity, and a comparison with the St Thomas's disability index. In: Roland M, Jenner J R (eds) Back pain: new approaches to rehabilitation and education. Manchester University Press. Manchester

Baltimore Therapeutic Equipment Company 1986 Operations manual for the Baltimore Therapeutic Equipment work simulator

Bergner M, Bobbit R A, Pollard W E, Martin D P, Gilson B S 1976 The sickness impact profile: validation of a health status measure. Medical Care 14: 57–67

Bergner M, Bobbit R A, Carter W B, Gilson B S 1981 The sickness impact profile: development and final revision of a health status measure. Medical Care 19: 787–805

Bettencourt C M, Carlstrom P, Brown S H, Lindau K, Long C M 1986 Using work simulation to treat adults with back injuries. American Journal of Occupational Therapy 4: 12–18

Buckwalter K C, Wernimont T, Buckwalter J A 1982 Musculo-skeletal conditions and sexuality, part I. Sexuality and Disability 5: 131–142

Cairns D, Thomas L, Mooney V, Pace J B 1976 Comprehensive treatment approaches to chronic low back pain. Pain 2: 301–308

Callaghan D K 1993 Work hardening for a client with low back pain. American Journal of Occupational Therapy 47: 645–649

Canadian Association of Occupational Therapists 1988 Position paper on occupational therapist's role in work related therapy. Canadian Association of Occupational Therapists, Toronto

Coleman D 1993 Leisure based social support, leisure dispositions and health. Journal of Leisure Research 25: 350–361

Cromwell F S 1985–1986 Work-related programming in occupational therapy: its roots, course and prognosis. Occupational Therapy in Health Care 2(4): 9–25

DeLitto A 1989 Subjective measures and clinical decision making. Physical Therapy 69: 585–589

DeRenne-Stephan C 1985 Industry and injuries: arena for occupational therapists. Occupational Therapy in Health Care 2(1): 127–134

Deyo R A 1988 Measuring the functional status of patients with low back pain. Archives of Physical Medicine and Rehabilitation 69: 1044–1053

Dunne W 1993 Measurement of function: actions for the future. American Journal of Occupational Therapy 47: 357–359

Fairbank J C T, Couper J, Davies J B, O'Brien J P 1980 The Oswestry low back pain disability questionnaire. Physiotherapy 66: 271–273

Feuerstein M 1991 A multidisciplinary approach to the prevention, evaluation, and management of work disability. Journal of Occupational Rehabilitation 1: 5–12

Fisher A G 1992 Functional measures, part I: what is functioning, what should we measure, and how should we measure it? American Journal of Occupational Therapy 46: 183–185

Follick M J, Smith T W, Ahern D K 1985a The sickness impact profile: a global measure of disability in chronic low back pain. Pain 21: 67–76

Follick M J, Ahern D K, Laser-Wolston N, Adams A E, Molloy A J 1985 Chronic pain: electromechanical recording device for measuring patients' activity. Archives of Physical Medicine and Rehabilitation 66: 75–79

Fordyce W E 1976 Behavioural methods for chronic pain and illness. Mosby, St Louis

Gallagher R M, Rauh V, Haugh L D et al 1989 Determinants of return-to-work among low back pain patients. Pain 39: 55–67

Gibson L 1994 Functional capacity evaluation: recommendations for use and provision in CRS, Qld. Commonwealth Rehabilitation Services, Queensland

Gronblad M, Hupli M, Wennerstrand P, Jarvinen E, Lukinmaa A, Kouri J P, Karaharju E 1993 Intercorrelation and test–retest reliability of the pain disability index (PDI) and the Oswestry disability questionnaire (ODQ) and their correlation with pain intensity in low back pain patients. Clinical Journal of Pain 9: 189–195

Gronblad M, Jarvinen E, Hurri H, Hupli M, Karaharju E O 1994 Relationship of the pain disability index (PDI) and the Oswestry disability questionnaire (ODQ) with three dynamic physical tests in a group of patients with chronic low-back and leg pain. Clinical Journal of Pain 10: 197–203

Guttman L 1976 Textbook of sport for the disabled. University of Queensland Press, St Lucia

Hanson C S, Walker K F 1992 The history of work in physical dysfunction. American Journal of Occupational Therapy 46: 56–62

Harding V R, Williams A C de C, Richardson P H, Nicholas M K, Jackson J L, Richardson I H, Pither C E 1994 The development of a battery of measures for assessing physical functioning of chronic pain patients. Pain 58: 367–375

Holmes D 1985 The role of the occupational therapist–work evaluator. American Journal of Occupational Therapy 39: 308–313

Hook T W 1985–1986 A private practice work evaluation unit. Occupational Therapy in Health Care 2(4): 59–65

Hsieh C Y J, Phillips R B, Adams A H, Pope M H 1992 Functional outcomes of low back pain: comparison of four treatment groups in a randomised controlled trial. Journal of Manipulative Physiology Therapy 15: 4–9

Hudson-Cook N, Tomes-Nicholson K, Breen A 1989 A revised Oswestry disability questionnaire. In: Roland M, Jenner J R (eds) Back pain: new approaches to rehabilitation and education. Manchester University Press

Hurri H 1989 The Swedish back school in chronic low back pain. Scandinavian Journal of Rehabilitation Medicine 21: 33–52

Jacobs K 1991 Occupational therapy: work-related progress and assessments, 2nd edn. Little Brown & Co, Boston

Jerome A, Gross R T 1991 Pain disability index: construct and discriminant validity. Archives of Physical Medicine and Rehabilitation 72: 920–922

Johnston M V, Keith R A, Hinderer S R 1992 Measurement standards for interdisciplinary medical rehabilitation. Archives of Physical Medicine and Rehabilitation 73: S3–S23

Kennedy M 1987 Occupational therapists as sexual rehabilitation professionals using the rehabilitative frame of reference. Canadian Journal of Occupational Therapy 54: 189–193

Kielhofner G 1983 Occupation, in Hopkins H L, Smith H D Occupational therapy, 6th edn. Lippincott, Philadelphia. Cited in Cromwell F S 1985/1986 Work-related programming in occupational therapy: its roots, causes and prognosis. Occupational Therapy in Health Care 2: 9–25

King P M 1992 Profiling the work-hardening therapist: education and experience. American Journal of Occupational Therapy 46: 847–849

Kremer E F, Block A J, Gaylor M S 1981 Behavioural approaches to the treatment of chronic pain: the inaccuracy of patient self-report measures. Archives of Physical Medicine and Rehabilitation 62: 188–191

Labbe E E 1988 Sexual dysfunction in chronic back pain patients. Clinical Journal of Pain 4: 143–149

Lehmann T R, Spratt K F, Lehmann K K 1993 Predicting long-term disability in low back injured workers presenting to a spine consultant. Spine 8: 1103–1112

Lyons R F 1987 Leisure adjustment to chronic illness and disability. Journal of Leisurability 14: 4–10

MacDonald E M (ed) 1976 Occupational therapy in rehabilitation, 4th edn. Baillière Tindall, London

McDowell I, Newell C 1987 Measuring health: a guide to rating scales and questionnaires. Oxford University Press, New York

Matheson L N, Ogden L D, Violette K, Schultz K 1985 Work hardening: occupational therapy in industrial rehabilitation. American Journal of Occupational Therapy 39: 314–321

Millard R W 1989 The functional assessment screening questionnaire: application for evaluating pain-related disability. Archives of Physical Medicine and Rehabilitation 70: 303–307

Niemeyer L O, Jacobs K, Reynolds-Lynch K, Bettencourt C, Long S 1994 Work hardening: past, present, and future — the Work Programs Special Interest Section National Work-Hardening Outcome Study. American Journal of Occupational Therapy 48: 327–339

Ogden L D, Wright M C 1985 Work related programs in occupational therapy: a renaissance. Occupational Therapy in Health Care 2(1): 109–126

Ogden-Niemeyer L, Jacobs K 1989 Work hardening: state of the art. Slack, Thoroughfare

Ogden-Niemeyer L 1991 Procedure guidelines for the WEST standardised evaluation. Work Evaluation Systems Technology, California

Peters J, Large R G 1990 A randomised control trial evaluating in- and outpatient pain management programmes. Pain 41: 283–293

Polatajko H J 1992 Naming and framing occupational therapy: a lecture dedicated to the life of Nancy B. Muriel Driver Lecture. Canadian Journal of Occupational Therapy 59: 189–200

Pollard C A 1985 Preliminary validity study of the pain disability index. Perceptual Motor Skills 59: 974

Richardson I H, Richardson P H, Williams A C C de C, Featherstone J, Harding V R 1994 The effects of a cognitive-behavioural pain management programme on the quality of work and employment status of severely impaired chronic pain patients. Disability and Rehabilitation 16: 26–34

Riipinen M, Hurri H, Alaranta H 1994 Evaluating the outcome of vocational rehabilitation. Scandinavian Journal for Rehabilitation Medicine 26: 103–112

Ritchie M H, Daines B 1992 Sexuality and low back pain: a response to patients' needs. British Journal of Occupational Therapy 55: 347–350

Sanders S H 1980 Toward a practical instrument system for the automatic measurement of 'up-time' in chronic pain patients. Pain 9: 103–109

Sanders S H 1983 Automated versus self-monitoring of 'up-time' in chronic low back pain patients: a comparative study. Pain 15: 399–405

Sharpe G L, Liemohn W P, Snodgrass L B 1988 Exercise prescription and the low back – kinesiological factors. Journal of Physical Education, Recreation and Dance 59: 74–78

Shaw S M 1985 The meaning of leisure in everyday life. Leisure Sciences 7: 1–24

Sjögren K, Fugl-Meyer A R 1981 Chronic back pain and sexuality. International Journal of Rehabilitation Medicine 3: 19–25

Smith S L, Cunningham S, Weinberg R 1986 The predictive validity of the functional capacities evaluation. American Journal of Occupational Therapy 40: 564–567

Strong J 1992 Chronic low back pain: towards an integrated psychosocial assessment model. Unpublished PhD thesis, Department of Psychology, University of Queensland

Strong J, Ashton R, Large R G 1994 Function and the patient with chronic low back pain. Clinical Journal of Pain 10: 191–196

Tait R C, Pollard C A, Margolis R B, Duckro P N, Krause S J 1987 The pain disability index: psychometric and validity data. Archives of Physical Medicine and Rehabilitation 68: 438–441

Tait R C, Chibnall J T, Krause S 1990 The pain disability index: psychometric properties. Pain 40: 171–182

Tollison C D 1991 Comprehensive treatment approach for lower back workers' compensation injuries. Journal of Occupational Rehabilitation 1: 281–287

Turk D C, Rudy T E, Stieg R L 1987 Chronic pain and depression, part I: facts. Pain Management 1: 17–26

Velozo C A 1993 Work evaluations: critique of the state of the art of functional assessment of work. American Journal of Occupational Therapy 47: 203–209

Verbrugge L M 1990 Disability. Rheumatic Disease Clinics of North America 16: 741–761
Waddell G, Main C J 1984 Assessment of severity in low-back disorders. Spine 9: 204–208
Watt-Watson J H, Graydon J E 1989 Sickness impact profile: a measure of dysfunction with chronic pain patients. Journal of Pain and Symptom Management 4: 152–156
White J, Strong J 1992 Measurement of activity levels in patients with chronic low back pain. Occupational Therapy Journal of Research 12: 217–228
Wyrick J M, Niemeyer L O, Ellesson M, Jacobs K, Taylor S 1991 Occupational therapy work-hardening programs: a demographic study. American Journal of Occupational Therapy 45: 109–112

7

Treatment issues – techniques for pain management

Activity engagement 117
 Description of the technique 117
 Rationale for the use of activity engagement 118
 Efficacy of activity engagement 120
Activities of daily living preparation (through training, education and equipment provision) 120
 Description of the technique 120
 Rationale for the use of activities of daily living preparation 122
 Efficacy of activities of daily living preparation 123
Relaxation training 125
 Description of the technique 125
 Rationale for the use of relaxation 126
 Efficacy of relaxation 127
Stress management 128
 Description of the technique 129
Rationale for the use of stress management 129
Efficacy of stress management 130
Coping skills training 130
 Description of the technique 131
 Rationale for the use of coping skills training 131
 Efficacy of coping skills training 131
Groupwork 132
 Description of the technique 132
 Rationale for the use of groupwork 133
 Efficacy of groupwork 133
Creative modalities 133
 Description of the technique 133
 Rationale for the use of creative modalities 134
 Efficacy of creative modalities 135
Chapter summary 135
References 136

This chapter reviews a number of techniques which have considerable value for people with chronic pain. Each technique is described, as well as the rationale for its use with patients with chronic pain. Its use with individuals with pain is illustrated by case example, and available information on its efficacy is documented. The particular techniques covered here include activity engagement, activities of daily living preparation (through training, education and equipment provision), relaxation training, stress management, coping skills training, groupwork and creative modalities.

ACTIVITY ENGAGEMENT

We begin with the technique which lies at the core of traditional occupational therapy practice, that of activity engagement.

Description of the technique

Activity engagement is the term given to the active participation of the person with pain in personally meaningful and life-relevant tasks.

Activity engagement is not a matter of giving the person in pain something to do to keep him occupied. Implicit in such a technique is the personal volition and choice of the individual to do that which he finds challenging, absorbing, satisfying or enjoyable. Task selection is something arrived at through collaboration between the patient and the occupational therapist, taking into account previous occupational roles, interests and abilities.

Rationale for the use of activity engagement

In order to enjoy good health, human beings need to engage in relevant activities. One of the hallmarks of living with a chronic pain problem is the tendency of the individual to disengage from normal activities, due to a concern that activity equates with more pain. As was noted earlier (Ch. 4), such inactivity results not only in the deconditioning of individuals, but also in the escalation of the pain problem. By helping patients to engage in purposeful activities once again, the therapist enables the patient to, at the very least, interrupt the escalating pain cycle, and at best, increase feelings of mastery and well-being.

A further rationale for helping patients to participate in meaningful activities comes from the work of Wynn Parry. Wynn Parry (1980) observed that participation in work was the best therapy for patients with the unenviable pain of brachial plexus avulsion lesions. Brachial plexus avulsion lesions result in a pain characterized by hot burning sensations in the hand, coupled with sharp paroxysms of pain which occur periodically (Wynn Parry 1983). From his work with a series of 108 such patients, Wynn Parry observed that early return to the community and to work was the best analgesic: 'It behoves the medical team involved in the rehabilitation ... to help the patient get back to meaningful activities as soon as possible' (Wynn Parry 1980).

Wynn Parry (1982) went on to suggest that such engagement in purposeful activity may act on the patient's central inhibitory pain pathway, via the thalamus, to the raphe nucleus of the medulla, to the dorsal horn cells in lamina 5 of the spinal cord, thereby acting to shut the pain gate.

Heck (1988), an American occupational therapist, has illustrated how, by engaging in purposeful activity, students have a higher pain tolerance to electrically induced pain than when they engage in non-purposeful activity. Such a finding supports the idea that intrinsically motivating activities help to make patients feel less pain (Heck 1988).

McCaul and Malott (1984) provided a useful review of the literature on distraction as a method for coping with pain. Distraction was defined as 'directing one's attention away from the sensations or emotional reactions produced by noxious stimuli' (McCaul & Malott 1984). Support was found

reducing distress in response to painful
...iewed considered the acute, experimental
...tudy examining the benefits of distraction
...al pain states. Some evidence was found to
...onal resources required in the distraction
...in reduction. To an occupational therapist,
...se – the more engaging the task, the more

...tressed that much of the available literature
...te pain settings, and that more research is
...benefits of distraction in clinical pain con-
...ful area of occupational therapy endeavour.
...ciple of distraction or engagement in tasks or
...has much appeal for those working with
...only to think of one's own experiences with
...of the patients one has worked with. Pain is often at its worst, or most overwhelming, in the middle of the night, when there are few engaging activities or distracting tasks.

A case example illustrating activity engagement need in the treatment of an individual with pain is given in Box 7.1.

Box 7.1 The case of Mrs J

Mrs J was a 54-year-old woman who presented to pain clinic with a 7-year history of cervical and lumbar back pain and bilateral leg pain. The pain began after a motor vehicle accident. Prior to her admission to pain clinic, she had undergone four spinal surgeries and two knee surgeries. Before her accident, she had worked full-time in the public service in a clerical position. She had been unable to return to her work post-injury, and was now on an invalid pension. Her husband was on a carer's pension. Currently, her day centred primarily around meeting her self-care needs. She rarely left her bedroom, except to visit health professionals. On such occasions, she was pushed in a wheelchair by her husband. In occupational therapy, we examined her daily time use, her goals, and her previous interests and activities. She expressed a general dissatisfaction with her life. She acknowledged that she now accepted that she would always have some pain, but she wanted to have it better controlled. When directed to look at what she would like to achieve with this 'new' life of hers, she was overwhelmed – she had not looked at achieving anything apart from pain relief since the accident. It was revealed in her leisure history that she had once been interested in art, and that she still liked to appreciate art. She decided that she would like to try her hand at art, and in particular, drawing and watercolour. This involvement commenced on a limited scale while she was in hospital, where she attended the occupational therapy department and started drawing, and made enquiries about art groups and classes in her local community, and continued on her discharge from hospital. At last report, Mrs J still has ongoing pain, but is now active with her art interest, and is secretary of the local art group. She has derived considerable enjoyment and mastery from her participation in art, in addition to the reduction of pain levels when absorbed in her activity.

Efficacy of activity engagement

Few studies have been attempted to measure the efficacy of activity engagement as a pain management technique, particularly with respect to clinical, chronic pain. Heck's study, for example, was with experimentally induced pain in healthy university students. Support for the technique in the clinical arena remains largely at the case anecdotal level. Clearly, there is a need for occupational therapists to become more active in this area, particularly as it relates so closely to that fundamental belief of occupational therapy. Of course, such a study will be difficult. How is such meaningful activity quantified and equated between subjects; for example, does 1 hour of guitar practice for one subject equate to 1 hour of swimming for another subject? How can the effects of any concomitant treatments, such as medication or transcutaneous nerve stimulation, be balanced out? Still, much research is warranted.

ACTIVITIES OF DAILY LIVING PREPARATION (THROUGH TRAINING, EDUCATION AND EQUIPMENT PROVISION)

Description of the technique

The occupational therapist needs to consider the individual patient's ability to perform daily living tasks in order to maximize the patient's function. When an impairment is found in the individual's ability to perform activities of daily living, the occupational therapist may provide specific training to enhance performance, advise on adaptive techniques such as good body mechanics or energy conservation techniques to enable completion of the task, and/or provide assistive devices or adaptive equipment to help in task completion (Nichols 1976, Tyson 1988).

Training

In training an individual to enhance their performance on an ADL task, the occupational therapist may need to consider the patient's sensation, muscle strength, endurance, range of motion, balance and coordination. A sensory problem often seen in patients with chronic pain is hypersensitivity. Such a problem will benefit from a desensitization program, where the therapist uses a sequence of graded and repetitive tactile stimuli (Scott 1983). Range of motion and endurance are also problem areas for many patients with chronic pain.

Range of motion. Encouraging active range of motion is important for those patients in whom only guarded movements, due to the pain or the fear of pain, are observed. This can be particularly encouraged by involving the patients in absorbing activities which require active range of the relevant joints. 'The use of activity for stretching is empirically based on the idea that a person involved in an interesting and purposeful activity will gain greater range because he is relaxed, not anticipating pain, is motivated to complete the task, and will be more likely to move as the activity demands' (Trombly 1983).

Endurance. With problems of lack of endurance, the occupational therapist would again engage the patient in absorbing activities. In particular, an activity which is moderately fatiguing would be chosen, with the patient required to participate for progressively longer periods of time (Trombly 1983). Rest periods would be built into such activities to enable metabolic recovery (Trombly 1983). Such principles can be applied to any manner of activities in the patient's life. A graded activity program would be set up to increase endurance, using increasing periods of activity, or alternatively, increasing frequency of participation by the patient.

Adaptive techniques

Body mechanics training is seen as particularly useful for individuals with back pain, although it has a wider application to all types of bodily pain. McCauley (1990) suggested that such training should include instruction on positions and movements which will not increase the risk of low back injury. It is important for body mechanics training to have an applied focus. Rather than just telling patients to lift with the knees bent, the occupational therapist will explore each patient's occupational tasks and instruct them, showing how good body mechanics principles can be applied to such tasks within the relevant environmental context. In such applied training situations, in addition to instruction, the occupational therapist will ensure that patients actually get to practise such techniques, thereby providing opportunities for the patients to improve their self-efficacy in the area of task performance.

Equipment provision

The provision of adaptive equipment has also been described as a useful technique for enhancing the function of patients with chronic pain (Strong 1986, Tyson & Strong 1990). In a survey of occupational therapists working in pain management in Queensland, Australia, I found that 40% of respondents felt that the provision of adaptive equipment was the most effective component of their treatment (Strong 1986). Adaptive equipment is equipment which assists a person to perform a particular activity more independently or with greater ease (Bell 1984, Tyson 1988). It may include such things as back support cushions, over-toilet rails, architect-style tilting desks, wheelchairs and long-handled dustpans.

Rationale for the use of activities of daily living preparation

Improving the patient's performance components such as muscle strength, range of motion, balance and dexterity are particularly important rehabilitation goals, given the deconditioning which may have occurred in the days–weeks–months–years since the original pain problem began, especially if the individual was initially managed as if he had an acute pain problem. Long-term rest and inactivity have deleterious effects on the human body and the human psyche, and even short-term bed rest has been shown to be harmful (Berde 1995). 'Use it or lose it' is an apt statement here. The occupational therapist will therefore engage the patient in a reconditioning program.

Instruction in adaptive techniques such as body mechanics and energy conservation is undertaken to enhance the functional gains that the patient has achieved by reconditioning. It is particularly important for patients to learn about correct body mechanics as applied to various activities of daily living. It is good practice to teach people how to use their bodies safely and maximally when performing the variety of activities in their lives. Energy conservation techniques help patients to plan a more efficient use of their bodies and their time.

The provision of adaptive equipment to enhance the patient's function is a technique not without its detractors. As indicated in Chapter 4, such provision of equipment would be seen by therapists working from a behavioural perspective as being a reinforcer of pain behaviour. However, having declared earlier that I do not follow a strict behaviourist perspective, I find that the prescription of *appropriate* (and here I place emphasis on the word 'appropriate') equipment can assist individuals with chronic pain to improve their necessary task performance. Let me use as an example a back support cushion for someone with chronic back pain. If the reader can think about a time when they attended a 2-hour event (for example, a dinner or concert) and sat on wooden seat, or a plastic chair or stool, a level of discomfort may come readily to mind (I am referring, in the main, to individuals without a pre-existing back pain problem). For someone with an existing chronic back pain problem, participation in such an event may not be worth the increased level of pain and discomfort. Yet participation could be made easier by the provision of a back support cushion. In a case such as this, I would clearly see the use of adaptive equipment as a means for the person to enhance their participation in activities of daily living, and not as a sign of pain behaviour.

We return to the case of Mrs J in Box 7.2, to see how she was helped to continue to participate in art activities.

                                                                FOR PAIN MANAGEMENT   123

                                  ox 7.1), I looked at energy
                                  as applied to drawing and
                                  ble for her involved her being
                                  t an easel placed at the correct

                                  upational therapy during her in-
                                  dergone a laminectomy 2 years
                                  iatica. Ms D had obtained good
                                  ed a nagging, constant, aching
                                  urned to work post-surgery,
                                  o the pain. At hospital
                                  While on sickness benefits,
                                  she spent much of each day
                                  e instrumental ADLs, but had
                                  g.
                                  vity tolerances – standing 10
                                  ing a simple 15-minute kitchen
                                  ecome deconditioned. A
                                  ith Ms D for the period of her
                                  activities for increasing
                                  g and walking were all
incorporated into the program, since they were all relevant to the tasks and duties of a
school. Tasks were chosen by Ms D in consultation with her therapist. The sitting task
involved computer use and desk top work, with the goal of 1 hour sitting decided upon.
A standing tolerance of 50 minutes was agreed to, with the task of a bench-top silk
screen printing project selected.
   In addition to Ms D working on her daily goals to increase her activity tolerances,
she was also given extensive instruction in good body mechanics, particularly as they
related to teaching tasks.

Efficacy of activities of daily living preparation

The efficacy of techniques to facilitate participation in activities of daily living has been addressed by various researchers. McCauley (1990) examined the influence of instruction in good body mechanics on the work performance of non-injured workers aged 14–19 years. She used a controlled study to evaluate the effectiveness of 1 hour of body mechanics instruction combined with two on-site individual instruction sessions on actual body mechanics used by subjects. Significantly better scores were obtained by the subjects who received the body mechanics training.

A Canadian physiotherapist (Palmer 1989) compared the effectiveness of two methods of bed transfers used with patients following lumbar discectomy surgery. The average time off work for the subjects was 5.5 weeks (S.D. = 13.2), and hence these patients could not be classified as having chronic low back pain. Nevertheless, it is interesting to look at this study since it evaluated the relative efficacy of two frequently used bed mobility techniques, these being side-lying to sitting transfers and prone transfers. No significant differences were found post-surgery between the pain intensity scores, analgesic intake and amount of assistance required by the two groups. Nor were significant functional differences found between the groups at a 3-month follow-up assessment.

Cohen and her colleagues (1994) undertook a comprehensive review of the literature which examines the effectiveness of group education programs for individuals with low back pain. Studies between 1975 and 1992 were recovered, with only 13 of these, judged by two blinded reviewers to have a quality of greater than 5/10, being subject to further examination. This number was further reduced to six studies. Only one study conducted with patients with chronic back pain showed a positive short-term effect of group education on pain intensity. Similarly, only one study with patients with acute back pain found an initial reduction in pain and sick leave duration. No clinically relevant benefits could be detected in any study at the 1-year follow-up. While Cohen et al (1994) stated that 'there is insufficient evidence to recommend group education for people with low back pain', they also pointed to the need for future studies to consider appropriate outcome measures, methods of education used, duration of education and the use of appropriate, multivariate statistics in data analysis. Cohen et al's (1994) paper should be taken as a clear indicator for us as occupational therapists to be proactive in such research endeavours. We return to this point again in Chapter 9.

Efficacy of adaptive equipment

My colleague and I (Tyson & Strong 1990) examined the effectiveness of adaptive equipment prescribed for patients with chronic low back pain who had attended a pain clinic over a 6-month period. In particular, we examined the level of benefit that patients ascribed to the equipment and the level of compliance with equipment usage as the two measures of effectiveness. We found that 87.5% of the adaptive equipment was in use, with 85% of it considered to be of some benefit to the patients (the equipment included items such as supportive chairs and cushions, dressing sticks and shoe insoles). The frequency of use of the equipment, and the perceived benefit of such equipment, were found to be significantly associated with the number of times the patients had been seen by their occupational therapist. Such a finding is not unexpected, given that an increased length of time spent with an occupational therapist may promote better patient education about equipment use.

Results of these studies provide some support for the continued use of education in body mechanics and the provision of adaptive equipment for patients with chronic pain. However, more research is clearly needed in this area.

RELAXATION TRAINING

The use of relaxation techniques with people suffering from various medical disorders has been advocated for many years. The work of Jacobson (1938) was instrumental in establishing the use of relaxation in medical practice, although the discipline of medicine was slow to incorporate relaxation methods into treatment regimes (Elton et al 1978). In recent years, however, there has been a growing interest in the use of relaxation and its place in pain management (Strong 1986, 1991).

Description of the technique

Keable (1986) has provided a framework for describing the various relaxation techniques. She speaks of physiological techniques, meditative techniques and hypnotic–suggestive techniques.

Physiological techniques

Grouped under the physiological heading are progressive muscular relaxation (Jacobson 1938), modifications of progressive muscular relaxation (Bernstein & Borkovec 1973), simple physiological relaxation (Mitchell 1977), and biofeedback (Turk et al 1979). These techniques involve an intentional focusing on the tension within the body. Progressive muscular relaxation and its modifications involve a deliberate build-up of muscle tension followed by its release, whereas simple physiological relaxation concentrates on joint and skin awareness. Biofeedback in the pain area is usually concerned with providing feedback about muscle tension via biophysiological instruments.

Meditative techniques

Meditative techniques include such techniques as Benson's relaxation response (Keable 1986). This method draws on observations of various religious meditative practices (Benson 1976), and involves the use of a word or mantra which is subvocalized with each breath out for a 20-minute period.

Hypnotic–suggestive techniques

Included under the hypnotic–suggestive category are autogenic relaxation

(Schultz & Luthe 1969) and hypnosis (Hilgard 1975). In many countries, occupational therapists are not qualified or registered to perform hypnosis. New Zealand is the one exception to this rule that I am aware of. In New Zealand, appropriately qualified registered occupational therapists who are members of the New Zealand Hypnosis Society are allowed to use hypnosis. Autogenic relaxation consists of self-suggestion phrases to help the individual to relax, combined with advanced phrases to help control consciousness (Abildness 1982). It involves steps to concentrate on heaviness and warmth in the legs and arms, the regulation of breathing and cardiac activity, abdominal warmth, and forehead cooling (Schultz & Luthe 1969).

Rationale for the use of relaxation

There are three main models postulated to explain the mechanism by which relaxation can assist in pain alleviation. The reflex–spasm model and the stress–causality model (Collins et al 1982) both conceptualize the pain relief mechanism in physiological terms, while the cognitive factors model (Flor et al 1983, Hendler et al 1977, Large & Lamb 1983) views pain relief in psychological terms.

The reflex–spasm model

This model suggests that in response to tissue injury, inflammation and subsequent pain, increased muscle tension occurs (Collins et al 1982, Varni et al 1980). Such tensing of the muscles is a protective, guarding reflex aimed at immobilizing the injured area and preventing further tissue damage (Ong 1986). A vicious pain cycle is then established, with pain producing muscle tension and spasm, and muscle tension and spasm aggravating pain (Kravitz et al 1981, Varni et al 1980). When increased muscle tension is prolonged, then muscle fatigue can occur, itself contributing to the pain experience (Ong 1986).

Using such a model, the aim of treatment would be to reduce muscle tension in the local area, thereby breaking the pain cycle (Collins et al 1982, Varni et al 1980). Relaxation is one method which can reduce muscle tension. Such relaxation should therefore result in a reduction in the EMG levels of local muscles (Collins et al 1982).

The stress–causality model

The stress–causality model postulates that a person responds to a perceived pain or external stress by undergoing a generalized physiological response, as seen in arousal states (Collins et al 1982). Local and general muscle tension levels therefore rise, along with other physiological parameters (Collins et al 1982). The aim of treatment using this model would be to assist the person to dampen down the arousal state, and to attain the relaxation response.

The cognitive factors model

The cognitive factors model is the label given to the model which postulates that relaxation methods alleviate pain through cognitive factors. Many workers acknowledge the importance of stress and anxiety in the lives of patients with chronic pain (see, for example, Flor et al 1983, Large & Lamb 1983, Turner 1982). Relaxation methods are seen as a technique to reduce general anxiety and to increase feelings of self-control. Treatment using the cognitive factors model emphasizes the importance of instilling stress-reduction and coping skills in the person with pain (Collins et al 1982).

The work of Phillips (1988) and myself (Strong 1991) gives some useful indications in support of these three models. Phillips (1988) has shown that the immediate effect of relaxation training for patients with heterogeneous pain complaints is a reduction in both the sensory and affective dimensions of pain. I also found an immediate reduction in the sensory and affective pain dimensions experienced by a group of patients with chronic low back pain after relaxation training (Strong 1991). These two findings lend support to both the sensory and cognitive models as explanations for the action of relaxation.

A case example illustrating the use of relaxation in the treatment of low back pain is given in Box 7.4.

Efficacy of relaxation

A number of workers have examined the efficacy of relaxation techniques, including two occupational therapists (Engel 1992, Engel & Rapoff 1990, Engel et al 1994, Strong et al 1989). Strong and colleagues (1989) compared

---

Box 7.4 The case of Mrs D

Mrs D's reaction, when I explained to her how relaxation could help her low back pain, was typical of many patients I have worked with: 'But my pain is a real physical thing, so how could relaxation help?'. Using biofeedback as an adjunct, I was able to demonstrate to Mrs D how relaxation could reduce real physical tension in her muscles. Once she had learned of this connection between relaxation and muscle tension, Mrs D became quite an advocate of daily relaxation practice. She found it particularly useful as a technique to use in the early afternoon when her pain seemed to intensify. The relaxed state of body and mind then helped her to enjoy the early evening and mealtime when her husband came home from work. It was also useful for those nights when she could not sleep, sometimes helping her to drift off to sleep.

the effectiveness of applied relaxation and applied relaxation plus EMG biofeedback used with patients with chronic low back pain. 40 female patients, with an average age of 49 years, were assigned to either group using an alternating procedure. At discharge, patients in the applied relaxation group showed a significant improvement in pain intensity, but this was not maintained at follow-up. On the pain rating index (a more qualitative index of pain), patients in both groups showed a significant reduction at discharge, with only the subjects in the applied relaxation plus biofeedback group maintaining this improvement at follow-up.

Engel (1992) and her colleagues (Engel & Rapoff 1990, Engel et al 1994), have examined the use of relaxation for the treatment of children with headaches. In addition to finding short-term benefits in such training, they recently found beneficial effects at a long-term follow-up of four subjects, 81 months post-treatment.

Studies comparing relaxation technique effectiveness by other workers such as Linton and Gotestam (1984), Lacroix et al (1986), Large and Lamb (1983), and Turner (1982) have yielded mixed results. Linton and Gotestam (1984), in comparing applied relaxation and applied relaxation plus operant conditioning, found that the applied relaxation group had significantly lower pain intensity over time, while the applied relaxation plus operant conditioning group had significantly better results on analgesic reductions. In comparing EMG biofeedback, relaxation training, combined biofeedback and relaxation, and no-treatment control, Lacroix and his colleagues (1986) found that all three treatments were effective in the short term (and better than the control condition), but the relaxation training condition was more successful at follow-up. Large and Lamb (1983) found that both a biofeedback condition and a control condition were effective in decreasing muscle tension in patients with musculoskeletal pain. Meanwhile, in comparing relaxation training, relaxation training plus cognitive behavioural therapy and a control, Turner (1982) found that patients in both active conditions showed significant improvement.

Taken together, these results suggest that relaxation is of value in pain management. However, it would be useful to have further research work in the area, to help clarify which technique is most suitable for which pain in which patient, as well as the ideal number of relaxation sessions and the long-term effectiveness of the techniques.

STRESS MANAGEMENT

Stress management has been mentioned as a frequently used technique by occupational therapists working with patients with pain (Strong 1986, Zelik 1984). Swann (1989), a physiotherapist from the United Kingdom, has suggested that physiotherapists might utilize stress management techniques for pain control.

Description of the technique

Stress can be considered as the interaction between the coping skills of a person and the demands of his environment (Spielberger, cited in Montgomery 1985). When a person feels that the demands on them exceed their resources, we talk of them as being distressed. In stress management, individuals learn about the body's stress response (the fight and flight mechanism), and learn to identify relevant stressors and the manifestations of excess stressors on their bodies. They are also taught how to deal with such stressors, using techniques such as relaxation, with and without biofeedback, assertiveness training, communication skills, goal setting and cognitive techniques such as thought stopping and rational thinking.

Rationale for the use of stress management

Given the pervasive nature of chronic pain, with the frequent 'entrapment' of the individual in a chronic pain cycle, people with chronic pain frequently face problems in many areas of daily living. As we saw earlier (Ch. 1), patients may have interpersonal difficulties with significant others, health care professionals and employers; they may reduce normal activities, so that their daily lives revolve around their pain and its relief; they may even be overwhelmed by feelings of worthlessness, helplessness and anger. For such individuals, stress management techniques can be useful, enabling them to identify more easily the particular stressors in their lives (as distinct from their global pain problem), teaching them how the stressors impact on their underlying pain problem, and helping them to cope with their particular environmental demands.

At the most basic level, teaching a patient how stress increases muscle tension, and hence aggravates the pain area, can be a big step forward – it can often be difficult to see the connection between seemingly non-physical demands or emotions and actual muscle tension. The patient can then learn a variety of muscular relaxation techniques to prevent such an increase in muscle tension. Additionally, once the patient sees a connection between a stressor and their pain, they may be taught alternative ways to deal with such a stressor. Such methods may include the elimination of the stressor from their lives (if such a solution is possible), or the use of mental strategies whereby the significance of the stressor to them is diminished.

The case example in Box 7.5 shows how this might be achieved.

Assertiveness training and stress management

Using assertiveness training as another stress management technique, Zelik (1984) has described how it can assist patients 'by decreasing their

> **Box 7.5** The case of Bob
>
> Bob was a 27-year-old man with a 4-year history of chronic low back pain with left sciatica. The pain began after Bob was injured in a fall at work. Bob was married, and had 2 children, aged 9 and 6. He was paid out by the relevant workers' compensation agency, and was now on an invalid pension. His wife now worked full-time, and he stayed at home. Prior to his injury, Bob had worked full-time while his wife was the full-time homemaker and child carer. One of the things Bob identified in therapy sessions as being a big stressor in his life was accepting that his wife was now the breadwinner and that he stayed at home. Each morning, when he waved his wife off to work, he was stressed. It came as no surprise to find that he reported the early morning as one of the worst pain periods. Once Bob realized the link between his wife leaving for work and the exacerbation of his pain, he was able to use a brief relaxation technique to keep his muscle tension levels down. He was also able to reframe his thoughts about his wife going to work and him staying at home. He acknowledged that his wife was enjoying working; she did not feel that he had failed her and the family each day as she left for work. He also began to consider the positive aspects of being at home. He was able to participate more in the lives of his children (for example, attending school activities). With the combined strategies of relaxation techniques and reframing, Bob was able to eliminate this particular stressor from his life. Such strategies did not take away his underlying pain problem, but they did help him to make a better adjustment.

emotional stress and lack of control in their environments caused by ineffectual communication'. Such training for patients with chronic pain can help them to express their needs and feelings more effectively and to problem solve rather than 'bottling up' their concerns (Zelik 1984).

Efficacy of stress management

Studies which document the efficacy of comprehensive stress management programs are few. Studies of components such as relaxation are more plentiful, and have been outlined in the previous section. Certainly, more investigation by occupational therapists into the effectiveness of stress management programs for patients with chronic pain is warranted.

COPING SKILLS TRAINING

Coping strategies have been conceptualized as 'a response to environmental and psychological demands in particularly stressful situations' (Endler & Parker 1990). They are the purposeful efforts which people make to deal with the impact of stress (Jensen et al 1991). For people with chronic pain, the presence of pain, day and night, over time, can be a very stressful situation (Strong & Large 1995). 35% of people with chronic low back pain suggested that the pain was the primary stressor in their lives (Turner et al 1987).

Box 7.6	Classification of coping strategies
Physical	E.g. medications, surgery, transcutaneous nerve stimulation, acupuncture and concurrent tactile stimulation (Fernandez 1986)
Behavioural	E.g. biofeedback, hypnosis, operant conditioning (Fernandez 1986)
Cognitive	E.g. imagery, coping self-statements, attention diversion, pacing and planning (Fernandez 1986, Strong & Large 1995)

Description of the technique

One way of classifying coping strategies has been suggested by Fernandez (1986). He suggested that we talk of physical, behavioural and cognitive coping strategies (see Box 7.6).

We have already described many of the behavioural strategies earlier in this book.

The cognitive coping strategies all involve trying to modify the pain by means of one's thoughts (Fernandez 1986). Imagery may involve the use of transformation, where the pain sensation is considered more as a dull ache, or imagery where one imagines the pain leaving one's body. Coping self-statements involve the use of positive self-talk, where one tells oneself that one can manage tasks, achieve goals et cetera, despite the pain. Attention-diversion techniques involve using mental strategies to focus attention away from the pain, such as thinking of a happy occasion. Pacing involves planning activities and scheduling pauses or rests within such activities. Planning involves an evaluation of the consequences of doing or not doing particular activities, and making choices based upon such an evaluation.

Rationale for the use of coping skills training

As mentioned in the stress management section (p. 129), chronic pain is a syndrome where, very often, individuals feel that the demands placed on them exceed their normal coping skills or resources. In therapy, we aim to increase the coping skills of individual patients to help them to meet the ongoing demands of living with a chronic pain condition. The case example in Box 7.7 shows how coping strategies helped an individual to control chronic back pain.

Efficacy of coping skills training

The use of coping skills training for patients with pain is a wide-spread clinical practice. Such training is usually given as part of an overall treatment package. Hence, while some studies have evaluated the effectiveness

> **Box 7.7** The case of Mrs E
>
> Mrs E was a 58-year-old woman with a 5-year history of chronic back pain, which began after a fall on a wet concrete ramp at a shopping centre when she had an armful of parcels. She had had no back surgery, but had continued to be plagued by back pain. Mrs E had developed good coping skills over the ensuing 5 years. In terms of behavioural strategies, she had learned to avoid body positions which aggravated her pain, and she had begun to belly dance as a way of exercising her muscles and increasing her flexibility. She also practised some relaxation techniques using yoga. She had adopted a number of cognitive strategies, by which she managed her life more carefully, and evaluated the consequences of activities before engaging in them. As she said, 'I have to prepare myself to do the things that I enjoy doing, whereas before I just used to do them'. The disadvantage of such planning is that it lessens the element of spontaneity in an individual's life. The advantage for Mrs E was that planning allowed her to gain greater control over her pain.

of overall treatment programs, few have focused solely on the coping skills training component. Most of those studies which have focused on the effectiveness of various coping skills have been drawn from an experimental pain paradigm (Fernandez & Turk 1989, Tan 1982), where healthy subjects (usually university students) have participated in experiments using the tourniquet method, immersion of the limb in ice cold water, pressure, or electric shock to simulate pain. These studies have generally suggested that coping skills training has some promise, but further controlled clinical studies are needed.

GROUPWORK

A Canadian team of physiotherapist and occupational therapist (Herman & Baptiste 1981, 1990) have provided a useful overview of groups and their benefits for patients with chronic pain. Coverage of groupwork will therefore be brief, with the reader referred to the excellent works of Herman and Baptiste for a fuller account of the subject.

Description of the technique

Groups for patients with chronic pain may take the form of therapy groups, structured groups and self-help groups (Corey & Corey 1987). Often, a combined structured group using group therapy processes is used. Such a group would focus on the specific topic of pain management, utilizing the qualities of caring, support, modelling, role playing, and confrontation (Corey & Corey 1987). Pritchard (1991), an Australian occupational therapist, has described how groups provide a useful medium for clients with chronic pain to acquire the necessary coping skills of relaxation and stress management. Herman and Baptiste (1990) have described the necessary ingredients of a pain group as positive expectations, opportunities for mastery and autonomy, and a willingness to change attitudes and thoughts. The particular pain control group run in the occupational therapy department at McMaster University Medical Centre has been described (Herman & Baptiste 1990). This program utilizes a 7-week, twice per week format for 8–12 patients. They participate in relaxation, learn about pain control methods and pain cognitions, and discuss personal problems, with group discussions, role playing, cognitive restructuring and homework exercises used to facilitate learning (Herman & Baptiste 1990).

Rationale for the use of groupwork

'Since maladaptive patterns of thinking, feeling, and behaving are common to chronic pain patients with diverse etiologies, these problems can be effectively addressed by group methods' (Herman & Baptiste 1990). Pain groups provide a safe, supportive environment in which patients can learn more about their pain, can gain more realistic beliefs about their pain, and can learn more adaptive coping strategies. They provide a vehicle for helping with behavioural change (Pritchard 1991). Self-help groups are also beneficial for skill maintenance and support with an ongoing problem.

Case example. The well described case example given by Herman and Baptiste (1981, 1990) is a useful one for readers to refer to here.

Efficacy of groupwork

One of the problems in determining the efficacy of groups is the frequent use of concurrent modalities. For example, in the groups described by Herman and Baptiste (1990), patients may also receive interventions 'ranging from neurosurgical interventions, nerve blocks and pharmacological management to biofeedback, hypnosis and psychotherapy'. Both Herman and Baptiste and Pritchard acknowledge the possible influence of such concurrent treatments. Nevertheless, they point to the potential and pragmatic value of pain groups. Participation in the group run by Herman and Baptiste (1990) was reported to result in 79% of patients obtaining some to marked improvement.

CREATIVE MODALITIES

Description of the technique

Creative activities include activities such as drama, art, music, dance, creative writing, and verbal activities (Leary 1994). In the pain area, the creative modalities of poetry, writing and art have been used by occupational therapists. An Australian occupational therapist, Nyhane (1991) coordinated a project involving participants on a pain management program where a book of prose and poetry, entitled *People with Pain Speak Out*, was produced.

Rationale for the use of creative modalities

Creative modalities offer the opportunity for individuals with pain to get in touch with, and express, their feelings, either general or specific, related to living with a chronic 'illness'. In the pain area, such opportunities to become acquainted with one's feelings can be useful for two main reasons:

- Patients with chronic pain may have difficulty in expressing their feelings. In some cases, alexithymia, which is the difficulty or inability to be aware of or to describe feelings, may be present. Here, expressive modalities can help patients to become more aware of underlying feelings. Once such feelings come to consciousness, they can be better dealt with.
- Creative modalities may be useful as therapy, with patients able to work through their feelings of loss, and may help with adjustment.

In Nyhane's (1991) project, creative writing was used to help clients to express their feelings and to educate others about what living with chronic

---

Box 7.8 The case of Mrs J

Mrs J was a 48-year-old woman with a 2-year history of chronic low back pain. Her pain had come on gradually without any clearly identifiable incident or trauma. Her occupation was home duties. Neurosurgical investigations had revealed no operable lesions. Mrs J was married, with 2 grown children who were now married with children of their own. An evaluation of Mrs J on the Integrated Psychosocial Assessment Model (Strong et al 1994) discussed earlier (Ch. 5), indicated that Mrs J had many of the features of 'an active coper with high denial'. She had a high desire for solicitude, a high reliance on medication, a high pain intensity, a high level of denial and a high use of coping strategies, combined with a low level of disability. She was mildly depressed. In individual therapy, Mrs J participated in a magazine picture collage activity. The magazine picture collage is an activity frequently used by occupational therapists in the area of psychosocial dysfunction (Sturgess 1983). 'Thus the value of collage is in uncovering emotions, problems, anxieties and psychopathology initially' (Sturgess 1983). Using the topic of 'a typical day', Mrs J produced a collage with a woman in the corner of the page, some distance from a flurry of action pictures which filled the rest of the page. She described her picture as a woman like herself left out in the cold, while all of life rushed by her. Her children were grown up and busy with their own lives, while her husband was busy with his work. She felt alone and miserable. Prior to the collage activity, Mrs J had talked in glowing terms of her happy and supportive family. The collage and her discussion of it provided the first tangible indication of some of the underlying emotional problems which Mrs J was facing, and increased the therapist's understanding of her pain, and her pattern of assessment scores. Pain was useful to her, since it resulted in her spouse and her daughters paying her extra attention. This information was very helpful in guiding further treatment with Mrs J.

pain is like. The case example in Box 7.8 shows the use of creative activity in guiding the treatment of an individual with chronic back pain.

Efficacy of creative modalities

I am currently unaware of any study which has systematically evaluated the effectiveness of creative modalities with pain patients. Anecdotal reports attest to their clinical value, but further research work in this area is required.

CHAPTER SUMMARY

In this chapter, an examination has been made of the use of seven groups of techniques which occupational therapists typically use to assist people with chronic pain problems. These techniques range from the very traditional occupational therapy endeavours of activity prescription and activities of daily living preparation, to groupwork, relaxation training, stress management, coping skills training, and creative modalities. For each group of techniques, a brief description was given, along with a rationale for their use. One aspect of the technique was then illustrated using a case example. Finally, the efficacy of the techniques was considered using the available literature.

It became clear from this overview that much work remains to be done in documenting the efficacy of these techniques in the pain management area. Nevertheless, I am comfortable in introducing them as relevant pain management techniques, both because of the limited research base and because of my own anecdotal experience and that of other occupational therapists. As with any techniques, not all methods will be beneficial for all patients. The occupational therapist is therefore required to make a thorough assessment of each patient with pain, and to carefully select the techniques most relevant to each individual.

These seven groups of treatment techniques can be used with individuals with pain in a variety of settings, ranging from the specialized pain clinic to the general hospital, paediatric clinic or nursing home. The use of such treatment techniques can be guided by earlier assessments of the individual's performance in the areas of self-care, work, rest and play (see Ch. 6). There may be other techniques being used by occupational therapists which I have not covered in this chapter – some therapists with specialized skills may be conversant with a range of other physical or psychotherapeutic techniques. Here, however, it has been my intention to cover those techniques used most frequently and most generally by occupational therapists for pain management. There are some specialized practice areas which do warrant further consideration and these are covered in Chapter 8, on special topics in pain management.

REFERENCES

Albidness A H 1982 Biofeedback strategies. American Occupational Therapy Association, Maryland
Bell F 1984 Patient lifting devices in hospitals. Croom Helm, Sydney
Benson H 1976 The relaxation response. Collins, London
Berde C B 1995 Staying in bed: harmful for your health? International Association for the Study of Pain Newsletter, March/April
Bernstein D A, Borkovec T D 1973 Progressive relaxation training: a manual for the helping professions. Research Press, Champaign, Illinois
Cohen J E, Goel V, Frank J W, Bombardier C, Peloso P, Guillemin F 1994 Group education interventions for people with low back pain. Spine 19: 1214–1222
Collins G A, Cohen M J, Naliboff B D, Schandler S L 1982 Comparative analysis of paraspinal and frontalis E.M.G., heartrate and skin conductance in chronic low back pain patients and normals to various postures and stress. Scandinavian Journal of Rehabilitative Medicine 14: 39–46
Corey M S, Corey G 1987 Groups: process and practice, 3rd edn. Brooks/Cole, Monterey CA
Elton D, Burrows G D, Stanley G V 1978 Relaxation theory and practice. Australian Journal of Physiotherapy 24: 143–149
Endler N S, Parker J D A 1990 Multidimensional assessment of coping: a critical evaluation. Journal of Personality and Social Psychology 58: 844–854
Engel J M 1992 Relaxation training: a self-help approach for children with headaches. American Journal of Occupational Therapy 46: 591–596
Engel J M, Rapoff M A 1990 Biofeedback-assisted relaxation training for adult and paediatric headache disorders. Occupational Therapy Journal of Research 10: 283–299
Engel J M, Rapoff M A, Pressman A R 1994 The durability of relaxation training in paediatric headache management. Occupational Therapy Journal of Research 14: 183–190
Fernandez E 1986 A classification system of cognitive coping strategies for pain. Pain 26: 141–151
Fernandez E, Turk D C 1989 The utility of cognitive coping strategies for altering pain perceptions: a meta-analysis. Pain 38: 123–135
Flor H, Haag G, Turk D C, Koehler H 1983 Efficacy of E.M.G. biofeedback, pseudo-therapy, and conventional medical treatment for chronic rheumatic back pain. Pain 17: 21–31
Heck S A 1988 The effect of purposeful activity on pain tolerance. American Journal of Occupational Therapy 42: 577–581
Hendler N, Derogatis L, Auella J, Long D 1977 E.M.G. biofeedback in patients with chronic pain. Diseases of the Nervous System 38: 505–509
Herman E, Baptiste S 1981 Pain control: mastery through group experience. Pain 10: 79–86
Herman E, Baptiste S 1990 Group therapy: a cognitive behavioural model. In: Tunks E, Bellissimo A, Roy R (eds) Chronic pain: psychosocial factors in rehabilitation, 2nd edn. Krieger, Melbourne FL
Hilgard E R 1975 The alleviation of pain by hypnosis. Pain 1: 213–231
Jacobson E 1938 Progressive relaxation: a physiological and clinical investigation of muscular states and their significance in psychology and medical practice. University of Chicago Press, Midway Reprint 1974, London
Jensen M P, Turner J A, Romano J M, Karoly P 1991 Coping with chronic pain: a critical review of the literature. Pain 47: 249–283
Keable D 1986 Relaxation training techniques – a review, part I: what is relaxation? British Journal of Occupational Therapy 48: 99–102
Kravitz E, Moore M E, Glaros A 1981 Paralumbar muscle activity in chronic low back pain. Archives of Physical Medicine and Rehabilitation 62: 172–176
Lacroix J M, Clarke M A, Bock J C, Doxey N C S 1986 Predictors of biofeedback and relaxation success in multiple-pain patients: negative findings. International Journal of Rehabilitation Research 9: 376–278
Large R G, Lamb A M 1983 Electromyographic (E.M.G.) feedback in chronic musculoskeletal pain: a controlled trial. Pain 17: 167–177

Leary S 1994 Activities for personal growth: a comprehensive handbook of activities for therapists. McClennan & Petty, Sydney
Linton S J, Gotestam K G 1984 A controlled study of the effects of applied relaxation and applied relaxation plus operant procedures in the regulation of chronic pain. British Journal of Clinical Psychology 23: 291–299
McCaul K D, Malott J M 1984 Distraction and coping with pain. Psychological Bulletin 95: 516–533
McCauley M 1990 The effects of body mechanics instruction on work performance among young workers. American Journal of Occupational Therapy 44: 402–407
Mitchell L 1977 Simple relaxation: the physiological method for easing tension. John Wiley, London
Montgomery B 1985 Coping with stress. Pitman, Carlton, Victoria
Nichols P J 1976 Are ADL indices of any value? British Journal of Occupational Therapy 39: 160–163
Nyhane C 1991 People with pain speak out. In: Australian Pain Society 12th Annual Scientific Meeting Program & Abstract Book. Australian Pain Society, Sydney
Ong K L T 1986 Handling the patient in pain. Physiotherapy 72: 284–288
Palmer M 1989 Mobilization following lumber discectomy: a comparison of two methods of bed transfer. Physiotherapy Canada 41: 146–153
Philips H C 1988 Changing chronic pain experience. Pain 17: 165–172
Pritchard L 1991 The use of groups for relaxation therapy and stress management as part of a multidisciplinary pain management programme. In: Australian Pain Society 12th Annual Scientific Meeting Program & Abstract Book. Australian Pain Society, Sydney
Schultz J H, Luthe W 1969 Autogenic relaxation, volume 1: autogenic methods. Grune & Stratton, New York
Scott A D 1983 Evaluation and treatment of sensation. In: Trombly C A (ed) Occupational therapy for physical dysfunction, 2nd edn. Williams & Wilkins, Baltimore
Strong J 1986 Occupational therapy's contribution to pain management in Queensland. Australian Occupational Therapy Journal 33: 101–107
Strong J 1991 Relaxation and chronic pain. British Journal of Occupational Therapy 54: 216–218
Strong J, Ashton R, Stewart A 1994 Chronic low back pain: an integrated psychosocial assessment model. Journal of Consulting and Clinical Psychology 62: 1058–1063
Strong J, Large R G 1995 Coping with chronic low back pain: an idiographic exploration through focus groups. International Journal of Psychiatry in Medicine 25: 361–377
Strong J, Cramond T, Maas F 1989 The effectiveness of relaxation techniques for people with chronic low back pain. Occupational Therapy Journal of Research 9: 184–182
Sturgess J 1983 The magazine picture collage: a suitable basis for a pre-fieldwork teaching clinic. Occupational Therapy in Mental Health 3: 43–53
Swann P 1989 Stress management for pain control. Physiotherapy 75: 295–298
Tan S Y 1982 Cognitive and cognitive behavioural methods for pain control: a selective review. Pain 12: 201–228
Trombly C A 1983 Treatment. In: Trombly C A (ed) Occupational therapy for physical dysfunction, 2nd edn. Williams & Wilkins, Baltimore
Turk D C, Meichenbaum D H, Berman W H 1979 Application of biofeedback for the regulation of pain: a critical review. Psychological Bulletin 86: 1322–1338
Turk D C, Miechenbaum D, Genest M 1983 Pain and behavioural medicine: a cognitive-behavioural perspective. Guilford Press, New York
Turner J A 1982 Comparison of group progressive relaxation training and cognitive-behavioural group therapy for chronic low back pain. Journal of Consulting and Clinical Psychology 50: 757–765
Turner J A, Clancy S, Vitaliano P P 1987 Relationships of stress, appraisal and coping to chronic low back pain. Behaviour Research Therapy 25: 281–288
Tyson R 1988 The effectiveness of adaptive equipment prescribed for chronic low back pain patients. Unpublished Honours thesis, Department of Occupational Therapy, The University of Queensland
Tyson R, Strong J 1990 Adaptive equipment: its effectiveness for people with chronic lower back pain. Occupational Therapy Journal of Research 10: 111–121

Varni J W, Bessman C A, Russo D C, Cataldo M F 1980 Behavioural management of chronic pain in children: case study. Archives of Physical Medicine and Rehabilitation 61: 375–379

Wynn Parry C B 1980 Pain in avulsion lesions of the brachial plexus. Pain 9: 41–53

Wynn Parry C B 1982 The 1981 Philip Nichols Memorial Lecture. International Rehabilitation Medicine 4: 59–65

Wynn Parry C B 1983 Management of pain in avulsion lesions of the brachial plexus. In: Bonica J J et al (eds) Advances in pain research and therapy, vol 5. Raven Press, New York

Zelik L L 1984 The use of assertiveness training with chronic pain patients. Occupational Therapy in Health Care 1: 109–118

8

Special treatment topics

Paediatric pain 139
  Assessing pain in children 141
  Types of pain in children 142
Geriatric pain 144
  Pain prevalence in the elderly 144
  Pain thresholds 144
  Pain management programs 145
  Treatment guidelines 145

Summary 146
Cancer pain 146
  Types of pain 147
  Assessment 148
  Case studies 149
Chapter summary 149
References 149

This chapter explores a number of special topic areas where occupational therapists work with patients with pain. While the two previous treatment chapters have relevance to the work of the occupational therapist in these special areas, there are additional factors which need to be taken into consideration. Hence the need for this chapter, which examines the management of paediatric pain, geriatric pain and cancer pain.

PAEDIATRIC PAIN

To think of children in pain is to tear at the heartstrings. McGrath and his colleagues (1992) commented that parents, children and health professionals all have a role to play in the management of a child's pain. Parents have the roles of experts on their children, coaches for their children and advocates for their children. Children have the roles of co-director of their management and experts about their pain. Health professionals have the roles of experts about pain management techniques, teachers for the children and parents, and caregivers (McGrath et al 1992). The occupational therapist working with children with pain needs to be mindful of these three functions. While much pain management for adults is organized through a centralized pain clinic service, most pain management for children is conducted in the general paediatric setting. McGrath and Unruh (1987) have spoken in support of the generalist approach, where all staff (including occupational therapists) learn about paediatric pain and its management.

The mention of pain in children leads immediately to the work of Anita Unruh, a Canadian occupational therapist and social worker, whose contribution to this area has been enormous. She and her colleague published the definitive book, *Pain in Children and Adolescents*, in 1987

(McGrath & Unruh 1987). Ronald Melzack, in his foreword to the book, commented 'McGrath and Unruh have performed a valuable service by dealing with one of the major problems in the field of pain ...'. The reader is also referred to other Unruh works on children's pain (Unruh et al 1983, Unruh 1992). Unruh (1992) chronicled the views on paediatric pain held in previous centuries, and found a reflection of the views now held about pain in childhood. Children do experience pain, and do require management of such pain. It seems that it was only during the first part of this century that the erroneous view was held that children are less sensitive to pain (Unruh 1992).

This section on children's pain is not a textbook. Rather, it highlights a number of aspects of children's pain of which the occupational therapist should be cognizant. It points to a number of areas of paediatric practice where pain is a particular problem, and it looks briefly at treatment methods. For a complete coverage of children's pain, I refer readers to McGrath and Unruh (1987), and the work of Bush and Harkins (1991) and Tyler and Krane (1990).

There are four common categories of paediatric pain (Varni 1984) and these are listed in Box 8.1. The occupational therapist may work with children with pain from each of these pain categories.

An important consideration when working with children with pain is the level of development of the child. Developmental level may have a bearing on the experience of pain, the measurement of pain, and the treatment methods used to manage that pain (Stevens et al 1987). In a study of 680 children aged 5–14 years, Gaffney and Dunne (1986) found a progression in children's understanding of pain which parallels Piaget's stages of cognitive development. Characteristic findings were that preoperational children (5–7 years) focused on concrete, physical aspects of pain, saying things like 'it is in your tummy' in completing the sentence 'Pain is ...'. Concrete operational children (8–10 years) illustrated a growing ability to think abstractly and a developing awareness of psychological aspects of pain, saying things like 'something that hurts you, you feel miserable and unhappy and you start crying with pain'. Formal operational children (11–14 years) were able to consider pain as having both physical and psychological components, as exemplified by

---

Box 8.1 Common categories of paediatric pain (Varni 1984)

Pain associated with trauma or injury	e.g., burn pain, orthopaedic pain
Pain associated with a particular disease	e.g., arthritis, haemophilia
Pain not associated with easily observable physical injury	e.g., headaches, recurrent abdominal pain
Pain associated with therapeutic procedures	e.g., bone marrow aspirations, injections

comments such as 'the way the body reacts when hurt' and 'a very hard thing to bear'. This study illustrated that children's understanding of the pain phenomenon changes over time.

Assessing pain in children

'Because children have relatively less experience, conceptual ability and social maturity than adults, their understanding of and communication about symptoms is often limited, (Zelter & LeBaron 1986). This will necessarily make the job of pain detection and assessment more complex, or at least different from adult work. (For a thorough account of pain assessment in children, the interested reader is referred to the works of McGrath and Unruh (1987) and McGrath et al (1985).) A number of novel methodologies for pain assessment in children have been developed. Such measures look at pain intensity, behavioural responses to pain and physiological reponses to pain (McGrath & Unruh 1987).

Methods

Oucher Scale. Pain intensity measures include the Oucher scale (Beyer 1983, Beyer et al 1983), which is a chart that uses a sequence of six photographed faces of children combined with a numeric scale from 0–100 to gauge pain intensity. McGrath and Unruh (1987) report that the Oucher scale has good psychometric properties. Alternatively, a series of happy-to-sad diagrammatic faces (McGrath et al 1985), or a thermometer scale (Katz et al 1980) can be used to measure pain intensity.

CHEOPS. In terms of behavioural responses to pain, a well known measure for postoperative pain is the Children's Hospital of Eastern Ontario Pain Scale (CHEOPS) (McGrath et al 1985a, McGrath & Unruh 1987). The CHEOPS looks at six behavioural areas; these being crying, facial expression, verbalizations, torso position, touching of the hurt area and leg position and movement (McGrath & Unruh 1987). It is a reliable and valid measure (McGrath & Unruh 1987).

Pediatric pain questionnaire (PPQ). Another comprehensive pain assessment developed for use with children and adolescents is the Varni/Thompson Pediatric Pain Questionnaire (PPQ) (Varni et al 1987, 1988). The PPQ also has a parent form for cross validation purposes. Dimensions tapped by the PPQ include pain intensity, pain location and qualitative aspects of the pain (sensory, affective and evaluative descriptors) (Varni et al 1987). Reliability between children's and parents' reports of pain intensity on the PPQ have been found to be high using correlation coefficients (Varni et al 1987).

It is suggested that the occupational therapist acquaint himself with the range of pain assessments which are available for use with children, and consider using some appropriate measure with children in pain. The use of an adult-type question such as 'describe your pain' may not be appropriate for the child you are working with.

Types of pain in children

Pain associated with trauma or injury

All-too-frequently seen here is the pain of burn injuries. 'Burns are amongst the most excruciatingly painful of injuries, and treatment procedures can be extremely adversive as well' (Maron & Bush 1991).

In addition to the pain, children and adolescents are faced with the issues of disfigurement and possible rejection by peers (Maron & Bush 1991). The use of a multidisciplinary team, which includes doctors, nurses, occupational therapists, physiotherapists, social workers and parents, is recommended for the total management of the child with burns. Comprehensive management of pain requires regular pharmacological management, relaxation training, supportive psychotherapy, cognitive behavioural techniques and behavioural techniques (Maron & Bush 1991). Building in distraction procedures such as cartoons during painful procedures can be helpful. While not suggesting that the extinction of all pain behaviour is the goal in burn injuries, behavioural strategies can also have a place in burn management. For example, Varni et al (1980) described how a shaping program resulted in the reduction of pain behaviours exhibited by a 3-year-old child who had been hospitalized for 10 months with severe burn injuries.

Pain associated with a particular disease

Healy (1991) has described how the occupational therapist can utilize guided fantasy techniques to assist children with juvenile rheumatoid arthritis to cope with the pain and discomfort of the disease and the pain of the treatment regime. Other aspects of occupational therapy involvement with such children would be the adaptation of self-care, play and school tasks to minimize pain and maximize function; for example, the use of clothing modifications to aid in dressing, the use of a light-weight computer keyboard for homework tasks, and training in coping skills. Attention to self-image issues may also be necessary to minimize the emotional pain of disfigurement felt by children with different diseases.

With respect to treatment according to developmental level, Healy (1991) found that for children with juvenile rheumatoid arthritis in preoperational and concrete operational stages of development, guided imagery techniques were most effective when incorporated into a story and play activity.

Pain associated with therapeutic procedures

There are innumerable therapeutic procedures children may undergo which can cause pain. They include infrequent immunization injections against childhood diseases, periodic dental procedures, postoperative pain, and the more frequent therapeutic procedures required by children with serious and life-threatening diseases. The child with cancer, in particular, may experience many procedures which are painful, including bone marrow aspirations, lumbar punctures, venipunctures and chemotherapy injections (Hockenberry & Bologna-Vaughan 1985, Lawrence 1994).

Multifaceted approaches have been recommended to assist children who experience pain from therapeutic procedures (Lawrence 1994, McGrath et al 1991). Strategies to give children information about the procedures they will undergo are recommended (Jay et al 1987). This can be achieved by role play using dolls and mini-props, filmed modelling or behavioural rehearsal. Children can be taught skills to manage the pain, such as relaxation, imagery and breathing techniques (Dahlinquist et al 1985, Jay et al 1987). During the actual procedures, children can be coached in using these techniques by parents or therapists, and positive reinforcement can be given (Dahlinquist et al 1985, Jay et al 1987, McGrath & DeVeber 1986).

Pain not associated with easily-identifiable physical injury

Two frequently occurring types of pain in this category are headache pain and recurrent abdominal pain.

Headache pain. The American occupational therapist, Joyce Engel, and her colleagues have examined the use of relaxation techniques with children with headache pain (Engel 1992, Engel & Rapoff 1990, Engel et al 1994). They found progressive muscular relaxation and autogenic relaxation to be effective in reducing children's headaches. Relaxation is clearly a useful component of a treatment package to help children with headaches. Lascelles et al (1989) have developed a treatment package for adolescents with migraine headaches which contains relaxation training, education in coping skills for stressful situations, thought stopping, realistic beliefs, assertiveness training, problem solving and imagery techniques.

Recurrent abdominal pain. 'Recurrent abdominal pain' is the term used to refer to at least three episodes of pain experienced over a time period of 3 months or longer which interferes with the psychosocial functioning of the child (Hodges & Burbach 1991). After a complete medical examination, behavioural and psychosocial assessments can be undertaken (Hodges & Burbach 1991). Although no specific occupational therapy literature addresses children with recurrent abdominal pain, the psychological literature supports the use of family-oriented, cognitive behavioural techniques including relaxation training, positive self-talk and reinforcement of well-behaviours (Sanders et al 1994).

GERIATRIC PAIN

It is my view that, like pain in children, pain in elderly persons has been a somewhat neglected topic until recently. It seems that at a clinical level, elderly persons have frequently been told: 'Well, what do you expect at your age?' or, 'You've just got to put up with it.' As Brochet and his colleagues (1992) commented: 'Very little attention has been paid to the occurrence of pain syndromes in elderly populations'. My own growing awareness of the problems of pain faced by elderly people was triggered by requests for advice from a number of occupational therapists working in nursing home settings.

Pain prevalence in the elderly

What then is the incidence of pain in elderly people? A French study looking at pain prevalence among 2792 elderly community dwelling elderly persons found that 68% had joint pain, 21% had severe back pain, and 22% had headache pain (Brochet et al 1992). 77% of a small Canadian sample (n = 56) of elderly persons reported having a pain problem (Roy & Thomas 1987). An Australian paper suggested that 20% of patients over the age of 65 years have a problem with chronic pain (Workman et al 1989). We can say that pain in the elderly is not an uncommon event. Yet Sorkin and his colleagues (1990) observed that 'few empirical studies have been conducted to determine the characteristics of the elderly pain population, their attitude towards treatment, or the effect of age on the ability to benefit from multidisciplinary pain management'. In this section, I will consider similarities and differences which may exist between older and younger people with pain, look briefly at assessment principles and overview treatment guidelines for use with elderly persons.

Pain thresholds

Some work suggests that older people have a higher pain threshold. For example, Tucker et al (1989) found that the cutaneous pain threshold (that is, the lowest point at which a stimulus first evokes a pain sensation) increases with age. We (Strong et al 1989) found that older men reported lower pain intensity on the Box Scale and the Present Pain Intensity scale of the McGill Pain Questionnaire (Melzack 1975) than did younger men or women of any age. Kaiko and his group (1983) found that older patients with cancer obtained better relief with less morphine than did younger patients. The exact relationship between age and gender and actual report of pain, pain threshold and pain tolerance is not clear. For example, it could be that in our study, the older men reported significantly less pain to me because they had been brought up to not show pain, particularly to a youngish woman therapist. However, one thing is clear about elderly people and pain – they are less able to deal with pharmacological agents.

Pain management programs

Two useful studies have examined the characteristics of pain in elderly persons and the reponse of elderly persons to pain management programs (Middaugh et al 1988, Sorkin et al 1990). Older patients were found to be as likely to accept and complete pain management programs as younger patients. Prior to treatment, they tended to use the same number of physical coping strategies as young people, but fewer cognitive strategies. They also had higher levels of pathology than younger patients and yet reported similar levels of pain severity, disability, support, affective distress and life interference on the West Haven Yale Multidimensional Pain Inventory to the younger patients (Sorkin et al 1990). The outcome data of 17 older patients were compared to 20 younger patients who had completed a multidisciplinary pain management program (Middaugh et al 1988). Despite pre-treatment differences on impairment (with older patients utilizing more health services and taking more medication), both groups showed significant improvement from the program, with older patients showing a greater reduction in use of health care services. These findings suggest that access to pain management services should not be denied to people because they are old.

Treatment guidelines

To recap on the sorts of treatments elderly people may benefit from in a multidisciplinary pain program, the program used by Middaugh and his associates (1988) contained medical management, occupational therapy, physiotherapy, biofeedback/relaxation and psychology. 'Occupational therapy focused largely on the use of proper posture and body mechanics during a wide range of daily activities to reduce the possibility of further injury' (Middaugh et al 1988). The medical input involved withdrawing narcotics and performing the necessary diagnostic procedures; physiotherapy focused on exercises; psychology considered stress management, pacing and cognitive coping strategies; while the biofeedback and relaxation sessions used progressive muscular relaxation, diaphragmatic breathing and electromyographic feedback. As we have seen in the previous two chapters, occupational therapists have skills in many of these techniques which can help the elderly person with pain.

In treating elderly patients with chronic pain, a number of factors may have a bearing on the patient and their pain. Issues such as the loss of spouse, social supports, home, income, health, mobility and independence may all influence the patient's suffering (Workman et al 1989). Such issues may need to be dealt with hand in hand with pain management. The use of a multidisciplinary approach is recommended (Workman et al 1989).

For therapists working with elderly persons with pain in nursing home or hostel settings, there is still much that can be done. Miller and LeLieuvre (1982) reported on a small nursing home study which examined the effectiveness of a behavioural program to reduce the number of p.r.n. (as requested) medications taken, the number of observed pain behaviours and the self-report on pain, and which aimed to increase the activity levels of four patients with chronic pain. Nursing home staff were involved in one training session explaining the use of reinforcement and extinction procedures. The patients then participated in an exercise treatment program. Unfortunately, the results from the study were not subjected to any statistical testing. Yet, the authors gave descriptive reports of a decrease in p.r.n. medication, pain behaviours and pain report.

Despite the absence of conclusive results, I suggest that this paper gives some useful ideas of the principles which an occupational therapist could incorporate into a program to assist residents with chronic pain. However, I hasten to add that I would not use such behavioural techniques in isolation from other treatments such as energy conservation, good body mechanics and the use of adapted tasks or equipment. Rather, I would incorporate such principles into an overall pain management program.

Summary

In summing up, occupational therapists can utilize many techniques to help the elderly to manage their pain problems better. Training in body mechanics, work simplification techniques, relaxation training, examination of relevant activities of daily living performance, engagement in an activity program, task adaptation and stress management can all assist elderly persons with pain. Additionally, depending on the setting, the occupational therapist may play his part in the education of family or staff about pain management principles.

CANCER PAIN

'Beyond the physical disfigurement and emotional ravages of advanced malignancy, it is the pain of cancer that is most dreaded' (Tigges et al 1984). Such a fear is not without foundation, given the prevalence of pain in cancer. Foley (1987) noted that, 'One third to one half of cancer patients in active therapy, both adults and children, and about two thirds of those with far advanced disease have significant pain'. In this section, I will look at the types of pain which patients with cancer may develop, pain assessment principles, general treatment management goals, and specific occupational therapy treatment goals when working with the patient with cancer pain.

Types of pain

Foley (1987) has identified 5 types of patients with pain, which are listed in Box 8.2.

She further defines cancer-related pain as being of somatic, visceral or deafferentation nature. Other workers have identified additional, non-biological pain of cancer (Driscoll 1987, Tigges et al 1984). Driscoll (1987) has identified psychological pain and social or environmental pain due to isolation or loneliness. Tigges and his colleagues have identified abandonment pain, isolation pain, and role-loss pain. I will now briefly look at each of these types of pain.

Biological pain

Somatic pain is a constant, aching, localized type of pain, due to things such as bony metastases (Foley 1987). Visceral pain is also constant and aching, but it is poorly localized (Foley 1987). It can be due to cancer invasion of organs such as the pancreas (Foley 1987). Deafferentation pain involves spasms of shooting pain on top of a burning pain, and is due to tumour invasion of nerves, especially of the brachial or lumbosacral plexus (Foley 1987). Management of these biological pains involves treatment of the tumours (as by radiotherapy), analgesia, adjuvant therapies such as antidepressants, nerve blocks, sympathetic blocks and neurosurgical procedures such as cordotomies (Foley 1987).

Psychological pain

Psychological pain may involve considerable depression and anxiety, and fear of impending death (Driscoll 1987). The treatment team needs to be

---

Box 8.2 Types of cancer-related pain

1. Patients with cancer-related pain of an acute nature (which can be both disease- and treatment-related).
2. Patients with cancer-related pain of a chronic nature (which can be both disease- and treatment-related).
3. Patients with cancer-related pain on top of existing chronic pain.
4. Patients with cancer-related pain in conjunction with a history of drug addiction.
5. Terminally ill patients with cancer-related pain.

alert to the psychological pain experienced by patients with cancer, and to be aggressive in its management, with the use of antidepressants, counselling, and active listening combined with specialist services of psychiatrists, psychologists, social workers and chaplains.

Pain of isolation. The pain of isolation and abandonment is often experienced by the patient with advanced cancer as family, friends and health professionals distance themselves. Such distancing often occurs when these people do not themselves know how to cope with the individual's approaching death (Driscoll 1987). The hurt experienced by the patient can be enormous. It is important for families and treatment teams to be aware of such distancing, and its effects upon the patient.

Pain of loss of role. Tigges and his associates (1984) have eloquently explained how occupational therapists have a special role in helping patients with cancer to deal with the pain of loss of role. The use of the occupational behaviour model discussed earlier, in Chapter 4, is recommended here. 'The goal of occupational therapy focuses on reducing the pain of loss of role by maximising the patient's potential to regain as many former roles as possible within the context of a very short future' (Tigges et al 1984).

Assessment

As with all pain management, a thorough assessment is necessary of the patient with cancer pain. A general pain history should be obtained, along with a measure of pain intensity, location and quality (Driscoll 1987). Measures used include the McGill Pain Questionnaire and the Visual Analogue Scale (Ahles et al 1984, Cleeland 1985, Driscoll 1987). An important consideration in pain assessment is the length of the pain assessment protocol. Many patients are not up to a lengthy pain measurement session or multiple sessions. The Brief Pain Inventory (Daut et al 1983) was developed for measuring pain severity, pain location and pain interference in patients with cancer. It has received support for its reliability, validity and sensitivity (Cleeland 1985).

A three-stage assessment for use by occupational therapists with patients with terminal cancer has been described (Tigges et al 1984). The need for such an assessment to be completed quickly and for treatment to be started early is emphasized (Tigges et al 1984). This assessment protocol uses an occupational history to determine the patient's past and present roles, choices and meanings, a temporal assessment to establish the patient's perspective on and patterns of time usage, and an assessment of the patient's physical status to evaluate sensation, muscle power, joint range, endurance, balance, coordination and mobility (Tigges et al 1984).

Case studies

Both Lloyd and Coggles (1988) and Tigges and his associates (1984) have provided illustrative case studies of occupational therapy intervention with individuals with cancer pain. Treatment techniques used by these occupational therapists included the provision of adaptive equipment, participation in activity sessions to increase activity tolerance, imagery and deep breathing exercises, energy conservation techniques, adaptation of tasks and assistance in implementing coping strategies. Such treatment by the occupational therapist goes a considerable way towards reducing the pain of loss of role, can reduce psychological pain and the pain of isolation and abandonment, and can also help as an adjuvant in biological pain control.

Of course, the occupational therapist is just one of a team of health professionals looking at the management of the patient with cancer. Further information on the general management of patients with cancer can by gained from the work of Tigges and Marcil (1988).

CHAPTER SUMMARY

In this chapter, an examination has been made of three special areas where the occupational therapist may work with people with pain, these being children with pain, elderly persons with pain and people with cancer. It is suggested that the additional, specific knowledge discussed in this chapter will maximize the occupational therapist's ability to enhance the patient's occupational performance and quality of life.

REFERENCES

Ahles T A, Ruckdeschel J C, Blanchard E B 1984 Cancer-related pain, part II: assessment with visual analogue scales. Journal of Psychosomatic Research 28: 121–124
Beyer J 1983 The Oucher Scale © University of Virginia Alumni Patents Foundation
Beyer J, De Good D, Ashley L, Russell G 1983 Patterns of postoperative analgesia use with adults and children following cardiac surgery. Pain 17: 71–81
Brochet B, Michel P, Barberger-Gateau P, Dartigues J F, Henry P 1992 Pain in the elderly: an epidemiological study in south-western France. Pain Clinic 5: 73–79
Bush J P, Harkins S W (eds) 1991 Children in pain: clinical and research issues from a developmental perspective. Springer-Verlag, New York
Cleeland C S 1985 Measurement and prevalence of pain in cancer. Seminars in Oncology Nursing 1: 87–92
Dahlinquist L M, Gil K M, Armstrong D, Ginsberg A, Jones B 1985 Behavioural management of children's distress during chemotherapy. Journal of Behavioural Therapy and Experimental Psychiatry 16: 325–329
Daut R L, Cleeland C S, Flanery R C 1983 Development of the Wisconsin brief pain questionnaire to assess pain in cancer and other diseases. Pain 17: 197–210
Driscoll C E 1987 Pain management. Primary Care 14: 337–352

Engel J M 1992 Relaxation training: a self-help approach for children with headaches. American Journal of Occupational Therapy 46: 591–596

Engel J M, Rapoff M A 1990 Biofeedback-assisted relaxation training for adult and paediatric headache disorders. Occupational Therapy Journal of Research 10: 283–299

Engel J M, Rapoff M A, Pressman A R 1994 The durability of relaxation training in paediatric headache management. Occupational Therapy Journal of Research 14: 183–190

Foley K M 1987 Cancer pain syndromes. Journal of Pain and Symptom Management 2: S13–S17

Gaffney A, Dunne E A 1986 Developmental aspects of children's definitions of pain. Pain 26: 105–117

Goodman J E, McGrath P J 1991 The epidemiology of pain in children and adolescents: a review. Pain 46: 247–264

Healy M L 1991 Guided fantasy: a method for teaching coping skills to the young child with juvenile rheumatoid arthritis. Occupational Therapy Practice 2: 40–50

Hockenberry M J, Bologna-Vaughan S 1985 Preparation for intrusive procedures using noninvasive techniques in children with cancer: state of the art vs new trends. Cancer Nursing 8: 87–102

Hodges K, Burbach P J 1991 Recurrent abdominal pain. In: Bush J P, Harkins S W (eds) Children in pain: clinical and research issues from a developmental perspective. Springer-Verlag, New York

Jay S M, Elliot C H, Katz E, Siegel S E 1987 Cognitive-behavioural and pharmacological interventions for children's distress during painful medical procedures. Journal of Consulting and Clinical Psychology 55: 860–865

Kaiko R F, Wallenstein S L, Rogers A G, Houde R W 1983 Sources of variation in analgesic responses in cancer patients with chronic pain receiving morphine. Pain 15: 191–200

Katz et al 1980 Distress behaviour in children with cancer undergoing medical procedures: developmental considerations. Journal of Consulting and Clinical Psychology 48: 356–365

Lascelles M A, Cunningham J, McGrath P, Sullivan M J L 1989 Teaching coping strategies to adolescents with migraine. Journal of Pain and Symptom Management 4: 135–145

Lawrence L 1994 Cognitive-behavioural management of chemotherapy injection pain in young children with leukaemia. Unpublished Honours thesis, Department of Occupational Therapy, University of Queensland

Lloyd C, Coggles L 1988 Contribution of occupational therapy to pain management in cancer patients with metastatic breast cancer. American Journal of Hospice Care 5: 36–38

McGrath P A 1987 An assessment of children's pain: a review of behavioural, physiological and direct scaling techniques. Pain 31: 147–176

McGrath P A 1989 Evaluating a child's pain. Journal of Pain and Symptom Management 4: 198–214

McGrath P A 1991 Intervention and management. In: children in pain, clinical and research issues from a developmental perspective. Springer-Verlag, New York

McGrath P A, DeVeber L L 1986 Helping children cope with painful procedures. American Journal of Nursing 86: 1278–1279

McGrath P J, Unruh A M 1987 Pain in children and adolescents. Elsevier, Amsterdam

McGrath P J, Johnson G, Goodman J T et al 1985a The CHEOPS: a behavioural scale to measure post-operative pain in children. In: Fields H L, Dubner R, Cervero F (eds) Advances in pain research and therapy. Raven Press, New York

McGrath P A, DeVeber L L, Hearn M T 1985b Multidimensional pain assessment in children. In: Fields H L, Dubner R, Cervero F (eds) Advances in pain research and therapy. Raven Press, New York

McGrath P J, Mathews J R, Pigeon H 1991 Assessment of pain in children: a systematic psychosocial model. In: Bond M R, Charlton J E, Woolf C J (eds) Proceedings of the VIth World Congress on Pain. Elsevier, Amsterdam

McGrath P J, Finey G A, Turner C J 1992 Making cancer less painful: a handbook for parents. Oncology Unit, Izaak Walton Killam Children's Hospital, Halifax, Nova Scotia

Maron M, Bush J P 1991 Burn injury and treatment pain. In: Bush J P, Harkins S W (eds) Children in pain. Clinical and research issues from a developmental perspective. Springer-Verlag, New York

Melzack R 1975 The McGill pain questionnaire: major properties and scoring methods. Pain 1: 277–299

Middaugh S J, Levin R B, Kee W G, Barchiesi F D, Roberts J M 1988 Chronic pain: its treatment in geriatric and younger patients. Archives of Physical Medicine and Rehabilitation 69: 1021–1026

Miller C, LeLieuvre R B 1982 A method to reduce chronic pain in elderly nursing home residents. Gerontologist 22: 314–317

Roy R, Thomas M 1987 Pain, depression, and illness behaviour in a community sample of active elderly persons: elderly persons with and without pain, part II. Clinical Journal of Pain 3: 207–211

Sanders M R, Shepherd R W, Cleghorn G, Woolford H 1994 The treatment of recurrent abdominal pain in children: a controlled comparison of cognitive-behavioural family interventions and standard paediatric care. Journal of Consulting and Clinical Psychology 62: 306–314

Sorkin B A, Rudy T E, Hanlon R B, Turk D C, Stieg R L 1990 Chronic pain in old and young patients: differences appear less important than similarities. Journal of Gerontology 45: 64–68

Stevens B, Hunsberger M, Browne G 1987 Pain in children: theoretical research and practice dilemmas. Journal of Pediatric Nursing 2: 154–166

Strong J, Cramond F, Maas F 1989 The effectiveness of relaxation techniques for patients who have chronic low back pain. The Occupational Therapy Journal of Research 9: 184–192

Thompson K L, Varni J W 1986 A developmental cognitive-behavioural approach to paediatric pain assessment. Pain 25: 283–296

Tigges K N, Marcil W M 1988 Terminal and life-threatening illness: an occupational behaviour perspective. Slack, Thoroughfare

Tigges K N, Sherman L M, Sherwin F S 1984 Perspectives on the pain of the hospice patient: the roles of the occupational therapist and physician. Occupational Therapy in Health Care 1: 55–68

Tucker M A, Andrew M F, Ogle S J, Davidson J G 1989 Age-associated change in pain threshold measured by transcutaneous neuronal electrical stimulation. Age and Ageing 18: 241–246

Tyler D C, Krane E J 1990 (eds) Advances in pain research and therapy, volume 15: pediatric pain. Raven Press, New York

Unruh A M 1992 Voices from the past: ancient views of pain in childhood. Clinical Journal of Pain 8: 247–254

Unruh A, McGrath P, Cunningham S J, Humphreys P 1983 Children's drawings of their pain. Pain 17: 385–392

Varni J W, Bessman C A, Russo D C, Cataldo M F 1980 Behavioural management of chronic pain in children: case study. Archives of Physical Medicine and Rehabilitation 61: 375–379

Varni J W 1984 Pediatric pain: a biobehavioral perspective. Behavior Therapist 7: 23–25

Varni J W, Bessman C A, Russo D C, Cataldo M F 1980 Behavioral management of chronic pain in children: case study. Archives of Physical Medicine and Rehabilitation 61: 375–379

Varni J W, Thompson K L, Hanson V 1987 The Varni/Thompson pediatric pain questionnaire, part I: chronic musculoskeletal pain in juvenile rheumatoid arthritis. Pain 28: 27–38

Varni J W, Wilcox K T, Hanson V, Brik R 1988 Chronic musculoskeletal pain and functional status in juvenile rheumatoid arthritis: an empirical model. Pain 32: 1–7

Workman B S, Ciccone V, Christophidis N 1989 Pain management in the elderly. Australian Family Physician 12: 1515–1527

Zelter L, LeBaron S 1986 Assessment of acute pain and anxiety and chemotherapy-related nausea and vomiting in children and adolescents. Hospice Journal 2: 75–98

SECTION 3
Synthesis

In this chapter, a synthesis is made of the material presented in the book.

SECTION CONTENTS

9. Synthesis   155

9

Synthesis

Review 155
Essential knowledge and skills 156
　The basics of pain　156
　Extent of pain　157
　Pain management models　157
　Occupational therapy practice models　158

Occupational therapy assessment　159
Scope of occupational therapy
　treatment　160
Techniques　161
Special areas　161
The future　162

REVIEW

As stated in the preface to this book, I believe that there is much that occupational therapists can do to help individuals with pain. This belief served as the impetus for the writing of this book. Rather than having each occupational therapist starting at the beginning and inventing her own wheel, I have aimed to provide a rudimentary wheel to guide occupational therapy practice with individuals with pain. Using this as the starting point, occupational therapists can focus their considerable talents and energies towards increasing the momentum and direction and accuracy of our wheel. Such implementation and refinement of occupational therapy practices can be only beneficial for individuals suffering from pain and its sequelae.

This chapter gathers together some of the knowledge and skills considered necessary for occupational therapists to work in pain management. These initially involve an understanding of the anatomy and physiology of pain: we must first understand what it is that affects our patients. From here, we need to be mindful of the epidemiology of pain, and of the models used in the management of pain problems. With this background, we then need to look within, to decide what it truly is that we as occupational therapists can offer to individuals with pain. It is my belief that what I as an occupational therapist offer to the patient with pain is a unique, special service. Having arrived at a model for occupational therapy practice in the area, and the delineation of the occupational therapy role, it becomes possible to direct attention outwards and forwards. This final section of this book tries to place occupational therapy in pain management within the context of the wider scene of pain management practices, and raises a number of issues and challenges which pain management occupational therapists will (or may already) face. Directions for future practice and development will also be suggested.

ESSENTIAL KNOWLEDGE AND SKILLS

To work with a person with pain, the occupational therapist needs to be intimately acquainted with the anatomy and physiology of the pain experience.

This point is crucial for the credibility of the occupational therapist – credibility with the patient and credibility with the other treatment team members. So often, patients have said to me 'But you can't understand my pain; you've never experienced it!' To which I can truthfully answer: 'You are quite right, I have never experienced pain such as you are feeling, but from studying pain for [x] years, I can understand that your pain may have the nature of a burning, shooting pain which is relentless in nature. I can appreciate some, but not all of the problems that pain has caused in your life. From this basic understanding, I am keen to listen to and learn more from you about how the pain has affected your life and to work with you to reach achievable life goals!' Such an honest response to a patient can be very reassuring, and can foster his active participation in a management program. In a slightly different vein, it is crucial for occupational therapists to have credibility with other health professionals. Etched in my memory is the meeting referred to in Chapter 1, between an occupational therapist, myself and two other professionals to discuss pain management and treatment offerings. My mortification at the occupational therapist's apparent ignorance of the gate control theory of pain remains. How can other professional groups give credence and respect to the occupational therapy contribution in such a case?

The basics of pain

With respect to the basics of pain, we need to know the following:

- Pain is both a physical and psychological experience.
- Pain is a complex phenomenon.
- We have a biological imperative to obtain relief from pain.
- Acute pain serves a useful biological purpose to the individual, while chronic pain does not.
- Chronic pain is pain which persists for longer than 3 months.
- The pain experienced by an individual may be modified (either reduced or increased) by factors such as past experiences, emotions, cognitions, and physical modalities such as counter-stimulation.
- The gate control theory of pain refers to this ability of the organism to modify pain perception at the level of the spinal cord dorsal horn via peripheral mechanisms or higher cortical descending influences.
- Chronic pain typically results in individuals displaying a constellation of problems affecting psychological, physical, vocational and social functioning.
- Pain is an anathema to the human being.

Extent of pain

Having gained an understanding about the nature of pain and how it affects the individual, the occupational therapist then needs to be aware of the extent of the pain problem in our communities:

- Chronic pain is a debilitating and expensive condition.
- In 1986, the cost of chronic pain in Australia was $7.8 billion.
- The cost of compensation claims for spinal disorders in Quebec, Canada in 1981 was $150 million.
- 81.7% of New Zealand subjects in a large epidemiological study (n = 1498) had had a pain experience.
- 32.6% of American adults in a large survey (n = 6913) had musculo-skeletal symptoms.
- 14.4% of American adults in a survey of 3023 adults suffered chronic pain.
- Low back pain is the most common type of chronic pain.
- Back pain typically has a recurring nature.
- Possible risk factors in the development of low back pain include lifting, forward bending, carrying, bending and twisting, monotonous work, work dissatisfaction, worry, fatigue, low fitness levels, low trunk strength, whole body vibration and smoking.
- 70–80% of the population will have a back problem at some point during their lives.
- 90% of these people will recover but the other 10% develop a chronic back pain problem.

Pain management models

Occupational therapists need to be cognizant of the current models for managing individuals with pain problems. Different types of management practices can be identified, for people with acute pain, chronic cancer pain, and chronic non-cancer pain, for prevention programs:

- Chronic non-cancer pain is best managed by the multidisciplinary or interdisciplinary pain clinic. Such an approach produces vastly superior results to sequential treatment by single specialists.
- Acute pain management requires a proactive approach which makes use of such techniques as pre-emptive analgesia, patient-controlled analgesia and continuous regional anaesthesia.
- Occupational therapists can assist in acute pain management in practice areas of burn management, hand therapy and procedural pain such as injection pain.
- The goals of chronic cancer management are to alleviate pain and control symptoms, and support the patient and their family.

- The central components of cancer pain management include the use of pharmacological agents, surgical interventions, radiotherapy, chemotherapy and hormone therapy.
- The occupational therapy role in cancer pain management was expanded on in Chapter 8.
- The goal of chronic non-cancer pain management is to rehabilitate the patient to an improved quality of life, regardless of the amount of pain reduction.
- Some pain clinics focus upon pain reduction whereas others focus on improving the patient's quality of life.
- The predominant approaches to managing patients with chronic non-cancer pain are:
  —the operant behavioural approach
  —the cognitive behavioural approach
  —the eclectic approach
  —the sports medicine approach
  —the functional restoration approach.
- Occupational therapists are often core members of multidisciplinary teams working with patients with chronic non-cancer pain.
- There is an important place for prevention and early intervention programs to prevent chronic pain problems from developing.
- Occupational therapists have a large role to play in both primary and secondary prevention programs.

Occupational therapy practice models

- For many years, occupational therapists have been involved to some extent in the management of individuals with pain problems. Such involvement has not been widely acknowledged or understood.
- Occupational therapists are concerned with maximizing the individual's functional status, and minimizing loss of roles and associated competencies.
- When working with individuals with pain problems, occupational therapists can be guided by a number of practice models, including:
  —the psychosocial model
  —the occupational behaviour model
  —the model of human occupation
  —the operant/behavioural model
  —the attitudes–beliefs–intentions–behaviour model
  —the appraisal model of coping
  —the commonsense model of illness.
- Utilizing a *biopsychosocial model*, the occupational therapist will address the biological, psychological and social aspects of the patient and his pain.

- When guided by an *occupational behaviour model*, the occupational therapist will consider the patient's competence in performing relevant self-care, work, rest and play roles, and will seek to maximize function.
- Applying the *model of human occupation* to practice in the pain area will guide the occupational therapist to consider the patient in terms of his volitional, habituation and performance systems within the context of the environment. The goal of intervention is to maximize the individual's occupational behaviour.
- One of the important therapy principles for pain management derived from the *operant conditioning/behavioural model* is the use of environmental reinforcers for well behaviours.
- The *attitudes–beliefs–intentions–behaviour* model emphasizes the importance of recognizing the attitudes and beliefs held by the individual with pain. Such recognition should be a central part of an occupational therapy approach.
- Gage's *appraisal model of coping* introduces the concept of an individual's self-efficacy beliefs and their relationship to coping with an illness or disability.
- Another important concept for managing pain is one's illness representations, as suggested by the *commonsense model of illness*. This model considers the individual's beliefs and coping strategies found in earlier mentioned models.

Recommended models

There is much to recommend in each of the above practice models. I have found it useful to be well acquainted with each model and to draw from it as required with each individual patient with pain. On balance, the two models which provide most guidance for my work are the model of human occupation and the attitude–beliefs–intentions–behaviour model. The appraisal model of coping is also influential.

Occupational therapy assessment

Having decided on a model to guide practice, it is essential for the occupational therapist to undertake a thorough assessment of the patient with pain prior to treatment implementation/management. It is crucial for such an assessment to be comprehensive and multidimensional, since pain is a multifaceted, multidimensional phenomenon affecting people's lives.

Aspects of the pain experience which need to be considered include:

- the pain description
- the individual's perception of the pain
- responses to the pain

- the impact of the pain on the individual
- how the individual deals with the pain.

We suggest that consideration needs to be given to:

- the intensity of the person's pain
- its location and extent
- its impact upon their functional status
- their attitudes towards and beliefs about the pain
- the coping strategies they use to deal with pain
- the effect of the pain on the person's affective state
- illness behaviour beliefs.

Such dimensions can be measured using our Integrated Psychosocial Assessment Model.

Assessments of particular use to occupational therapists include:

- *Performance systems measures* such as the Pain Disability Index, the Oswestry Low Back Pain Disability Index, muscle testing and functional capacity evaluation.
- *Habituation system measures* such as the Occupational History and the Activity Diary.
- *Volitional system measures* such as the NPI Interest Checklist and Self-Efficacy Gauge.

Scope of occupational therapy treatment

The scope of occupational therapy treatment will cover the individual's relevant performance dimensions of activities of daily living, work and leisure.

ADLs

One of the hallmarks of living with chronic pain for many individuals is a reduction in function in the areas of instrumental activities of daily living, personal activities of daily living, sexual activity, work activities and leisure activities.

Occupational therapy intervention may focus on increasing the individual's capacities (such as improved strength and tolerance), educating the person and/or modifying the tasks and environment.

Focus is also given to the individual's volitional system:

- What are their goals and are such goals compatible with performance capacities?
- Has the ongoing pain influenced their affective state?

Therapy efforts here are aimed at assisting the individual to adjust to living with chronic pain.

Work

The person with pain typically faces some disruption to vocational tasks. When considering an individual's ability to work, the occupational therapist may be involved in functional capacity evaluation, work capacity evaluation, work tolerance screening, work hardening, job analysis, on-the-job assessment, job site/worker modifications and job skills training.

Leisure

Leisure is an often overlooked facet of an individual's life which can also be affected by the pain problem. The occupational therapist can be of assistance here for individuals with pain.

Techniques

Techniques frequently used by occupational therapists with patients with chronic pain include activity engagement, activities of daily living preparation, relaxation training, stress management, coping skills training, groupwork and creative modalities.

Special areas

In addition to the occupational therapist seeing people with pain problems in a pain clinic setting, occupational therapists may work in the special areas of paediatric pain, geriatric pain and cancer pain. Of course, in general practice and specialty practices such as hand rehabilitation, occupational therapists will also encounter individuals with pain.

Paediatric pain

Children do experience pain and need pain management services. A child's understanding of pain, and their ability to express it will be dependent on factors such as developmental level.

Occupational therapists need to engage the children and their parents in the pain management process.

There are sufficient available techniques to gauge the level of pain experienced by children.

Pain can be experienced by children from trauma or injury, particular disease states, and certain therapeutic procedures, as well as some less easily identifiable conditions.

Geriatric pain

Elderly persons also experience pain, and as such, need pain management services.

Cancer pain

Pain is frequently found in individuals with cancer, and needs to be managed appropriately.

A well identified occupational therapy role with patients with cancer is assisting them to deal with the loss of role.

The occupational behaviour model has been proposed to underpin this work with individuals with cancer.

THE FUTURE

At this stage in our understanding of pain, it must be recognized that many people will have pain problems which we cannot relieve, no matter how hard we try and how often we try.

It would seem that occupational therapists have an important role to play in assisting the many individuals with pain problems to adjust to living with an ongoing problem.

Given occupational therapists' skills in helping individuals cope with illness or disability, there is much we can do in the pain area. Such intervention may occur in many settings, ranging from general services to special services such as cancer units, pain clinics and paediatric facilities, and with persons of all ages (since pain affects babies, children, adolescents, adults and elderly persons).

Currently, occupational therapy involvement in pain management could be described as patchy. While most pain services routinely employ, for example, a physiotherapist, such is not the case for occupational therapy. And yet the potential contribution to be made by the occupational therapist is enormous. Such a lack of routine occupational therapy involvement may stem in part from resource decisions. If a facility such as a hospital has few occupational therapists, then pain work may be seen as a lower priority than more traditional practice areas such as neurologic rehabilitation. It may also stem from that inherent difficulty in making explicit what occupational therapists 'do' for patients. If we cannot make it explicit, how then are we to convince our colleagues who make staffing decisions about the need for us on their pain services?

It is my view that occupational therapists, armed with a clear view of the contribution they can make to improving the quality of life of many individuals with pain problems, must be advocates of those individuals. Guided by a clear practice model, we must market our services accordingly. Such is one of the challenges we face.

Marketing of occupational therapy services for people with pain may occur in a number of ways. The International Association for the Study of Pain's Pain Curriculum for Occupational Therapists and Physiotherapists is an enormous advance. This prestigious international body has recognized the importance of occupational therapy in the area of pain management practice.

As we have seen, many methods of treatment for patients with pain remain unvalidated. Here is a unique opportunity for occupational therapy research endeavours. Does engagement of this patient in this particular treatment improve his quality of life? Does my education program on back care translate into change in vivo? Questions to which research can provide answers are seemingly boundless, giving the busy clinician or avid researcher a wide range of opportunities to evaluate practice. My own group is currently examining a range of topics, including the effectiveness of treatment in reducing pain and distress in children undergoing chemotherapy injections, the influence of family support on patients coping with pain, and the effectiveness of a back rehabilitation program on improving functioning of individuals.

Another marketing opportunity for occupational therapists may be in involvement in the local, national and international pain associations. Currently, we occupational therapists are poorly represented in such organizations. Become involved!

I would urge occupational therapists to consider what they can do in this exciting practice area.

Index

24-hour log, 83–84

A

A-beta fibres (type I AMH nociceptors), 9
A-delta fibres (type II AMH nociceptors), 9
Abdominal pain, recurrent, 143–144
Activities of daily living
  assessment, 82, 93
  instrumental, 82, 93, 99
  interventions, 160–161
  personal, 82, 93
  preparation, 120–125
  training, 120–121
  see also Function
Activity
  diaries, 85, 96
  engagement, 117–120
  purposeful, 49
Acute pain, 5–6
  management models, 31, 157
  occupational therapist's role, 31
Adaptive techniques, 121, 122
Aetiology, 22–23
  see also Risk factors
Alexithymia, 134
Analgesia
  continuous regional, 31
  patient-controlled, 31
  pre-emptive, 31
  WHO analgesic ladder, 32
Appraisal model of coping, 63–64, 159
Assertiveness training, 129–130
Assessment, 71–90, 159–160
  functional, 93–97
  habituation system, 82–85, 160
  models, 76–80
  paediatric pain, 141–142
  performance system, 82, 160
  reliability, 81,
  utility, 81
  validity, 81
  volitional system, 85–86, 160
  work assessment, 97
  worksite, 107
Attention-diversion techniques, 131
Attitude–beliefs–intentions–behaviour model, 61–63, 159
Australia
  Australian Pain Society, 44
  occupational therapy role, 47
  pain surveys, 16
Autogenic relaxation, 125–126

B

Back pain
  adaptive equipment, 122, 124–125
  disability, 24
  focus groups, 75
  group education programs, 124
  natural history, 21, 23–24
  New Zealand, 17–18
  nursing-related, 17–18, 38
  risk factors, 15, 22–23, 37
  Scandinavia, 19
  sexual problems, 98–99
  United States of America, 20, 48
  and work, 101
  work related
    New Zealand, 17
    prevention, 24, 37
    rehabilitation, 108–109
    risk factors, 15, 22–23, 37
Back schools, 37
Bed transfers, 123–124
Behavioural strategies, 34–35
  children with burns, 142
Benign cycles, 58
Benson's relaxation response, 125
Biofeedback, 125
Biological pain, 147
Biopsychosocial assessment model, 78–80
Biopsychosocial model, 51–52, 158
Body mechanics training, 123
Box Scale, 144
Brachial plexus avulsion lesions, 118
Brief Pain Inventory, 148
Burns, children, 142

C

C fibres (polymodal nociceptors), 9
Canada, 16–17
Cancer pain, 7, 146–149
  assessment, 148
  biological, 147
  case studies, 149
  management, 32–33, 157–158
  occupational therapist's role, 33, 162
  pain of isolation, 148
  psychological, 147–148
  surgical interventions, 32–33
  types of pain, 147–148
  WHO analgesic ladder, 31
Children in pain *see* Paediatric pain
Children's Hospital of Eastern Ontario Pain Scale (CHEOPS), 141
Chronic Disability Index, 79, 94
Chronic (non-cancer) pain, 5–7
  aetiological features, 22–23
  Australia, 16
  cancer pain *see* Cancer pain
  characteristics, 6
  cycle, 53–54
  and model of human occupation, 58
  definition, 6, 14
  epidemiology, 13–25

Chronic (non-cancer) pain, *Cont'd*
  management, 31–36, 157–158
  multidisciplinary approach, 29–30
  opioids, 32
  prevention *see* Prevention
  United States of America, 20
  and work, 101
Cognitive behavioural approaches, 34–35
Cognitive coping strategies, 131
Cognitive factors model of relaxation, 127
Commonsense model of illness, 64–65, 159
Compensation costs, 17
Coping
  appraisal model, 63–64, 159
  self-statements, 131
  skills training, 130–132
  strategies, classification, 131
Coping Strategy Questionnaire, 74
Cordotomy, 32–33
Creative modalities, 133–135

D

Deafferentation pain, 7, 147
Definitions
  chronic pain, 6, 14
  disability, 97
  pain management facilities, 30–31
  pain, 4–5, 14–15
Depression
  cancer pain, 147–148
  and disability, 96
Desensitization, 120
Disability
  back-pain-related, 24
  definition, 97
  and depression, 96
  types, 97–99
Disfigurement, 142
Distraction, 118–119
Downtime measurement, 96
Dual practice, 50
Dysfunction *see* Disability

E

Eclectic rehabilitation approaches, 35
Elderly people in pain, 144–146, 162
Endurance training, 121
Epidemiology, 13–25
Equipment, adaptive, 121, 122, 124–125

F

Fibromyalgia, 19
Function, 93–99
  measuring, 93–97
  observation, 96
  physical parameters, assessment, 97
  see also Activities of daily living

Functional capacity evaluation (FCE), 104
Functional restoration approach, 36

G

Gate control theory of pain, 9–10
Geriatric pain, 144–146, 162
Great Britain *see* United Kingdom
Group education programs, 124
Groupwork, 132–133

H

Habituation, 56–57
Habituation systems, 82–85, 160
Headache, 5
  children, 143
Health and Nutrition Examination Survey (HANES), 19–20
HIV infection, 49
Human occupation model, 56–59
Hypersensitivity desensitization, 120
Hypnosis, 126
Hypnotic-suggestive techniques, 125–126

I

Illness Behaviour Questionnaire, 79
Imagery, 131
Incidence, 15, 23
Instrumental activities of daily living (IADLs), 82, 93, 99
Integrated Pain Assessment Model (IPAM), 78
Integrated psychosocial assessment model, 75–76, 160
International Association for the Study of Pain (IASP)
  definitions
    acute and chronic pain, 6, 14
    pain, 4, 14
    pain management facilities, 30–31
  occupational therapy membership, 44
Isolation, pain of, 148

J

Job analysis, 106
Juvenile rheumatoid arthritis, 142

K

Knowledge-base, 156–162

L

Leisure activities, 109–111, 161
Literature, occupational therapy, 44–51
Loss of role, 148
Low back pain *see* Back pain

M

McGill Pain Questionnaire, 74, 144, 148
Management
  acute pain, 31, 157
  cancer pain, 32–33, 157–158
  chronic pain, 31–36, 157–158
  cognitive behavioural approaches, 34–35
  eclectic rehabilitation approaches, 35
  elderly people, 145–146
  facilities, 30–31
  functional restoration approach, 36
  models, 29–38, 51–67, 157–158
  multidisciplinary approach see
    Multidisciplinary approach
  multimodal approaches, 35
  non-cancer pain, 31–36, 157–158
  occupational therapy goals, 46–47
  occupational therapy involvement, 43–67
  occupational therapy role, 48–49
  operant behavioural approaches, 34, 60–61, 159
  postoperative pain, 31
  purposeful activities, 49
  scope, 160–161
  sports medicine approach, 35
  stress management, 128–130
  techniques, 117–135, 161
Marketing opportunities, 162–163
Meditative techniques, 125
Migraine, 143
Model of human occupation, 56–59, 159
Modified Somatic Perceptions
    Questionnaire, 79
Morphine, 33
Movement and Pain Perceptions Scale
    (MAPPS), 87
Multidimensional Pain Inventory (MPI), 76–78
Multidisciplinary approach, 29–30
  children with burns, 142
  efficacy, 36
  occupational therapy involvement, 43
Multilevel Pain Context Model, 80
Multimodal approaches, 35
Muscle tension, 126–127
Musculoskeletal pain, 19–20

N

Natural history of pain, 15, 21–22, 23–24
Neuromas, 7
Neuropathic pain, 7
Neuropsychiatric Institute (NPI) Interest
    Checklist, 86
Neurosurgical techniques, 32–33
New Zealand, 17–18
  hypnosis, 126
  New Zealand Pain Society, 44

Nociceptive pain, 7, 9
Non-cancer pain see Chronic (non-cancer)
    pain
Nuprin Pain Report, 20
Nursing homes, 146

O

Observation, 96
Occupational behaviour model, 52–56, 159
Occupational history, 84–85
Occupational performance history
    interview, 84–85
Occupational therapy practice
  dual practice, 50
  models, 51–67, 158–159
Operant conditioning/behavioural model,
    34, 60–61, 159
Opioids
  non-cancer pain, 32
  postoperative pain, 31
Oswestry Low Back Pain Disability
    Questionnaire (OLBPDQ), 82, 95
Oucher Scale, 141
Outcome expectations, 64

P

Pacing, 131
Paediatric pain, 139–144, 161
Paediatric pain questionnaire (PPQ), 141
Pain
  abdominal, 143–144
  acute see Acute pain
  assessment see Assessment
  associations, 44
  back pain see Back pain
  basic facts, 156
  behaviours, 34
  beliefs, 74
  biological, 147
  cancer see Cancer pain
  chronic see Chronic (non-cancer) pain
  clinical pain states, 7–8
  clinics
    aims, 33
    definitions, 30–31
    occupational therapy role, 49–50
    occupational therapy involvement, 45
  deafferentation, 7, 147
  definitions, 4–5, 14–15
  descriptors, 74
  dimensions, 73–76
  extent of problem, 157
  gate control theory, 9–10
  groups, 132–133
  incidence, 15, 23
  of isolation, 148

Pain, Cont'd
  management see Management
  modified gate control theory, 10
  musculoskeletal, 19–20
  natural history, 15, 21–22, 23–24
  neuropathic, 7
  nociceptive, 7, 9
  paediatric see Paediatric pain
  perceptions see Perceptions of pain
  peripheral, 7
  persistent see Persistent pain
  prevalence see Prevalence
  prognosis, 15
  psychogenic (idiopathic), 7–8
  psychological, 147–148
  risk factors see Risk factors
  somatic, 147
  surveys, 14, 15–21
    Australia, 16
    Canada, 16–17
    New Zealand, 17–18
    Scandinavia, 18–19
    United Kingdom, 17
    United States of America, 19–21
  sympathetically maintained, 7
  thresholds, 144–145
  visceral, 147
Pain Beliefs and Perceptions Inventory (PBPI), 86
Pain Disability Index, 82, 94, 95, 111
Pain Self Efficacy Questionnaire (PSEQ), 87
Perceptions of pain, 8–10
  measurement, 73–75
Percutaneous cervical cordotomy, 32–33
Performance, 57
Performance systems, 82, 160
Peripheral pain, 7
Persistent pain
  Canada, 16
  Scandinavia, 18
Personal activities of daily living (PADLs), 82, 93
Physiological relaxation, 125
Planning (coping strategy), 131
Postoperative pain
  CHEOPS scale, 141
  management, 31
Present Pain Intensity Scale, 144
Prevalence, 15
  Canada, 16
Prevention, 24
  occupational therapist's role, 24–25, 38
  primary, 37
  programs, 36–38
  secondary, 37–38
Prognosis, 15
Progressive muscular relaxation, 125
Psychogenic (idiopathic) pain, 7–8
Psychological pain, 147–148

Purposeful activities, 49

Q

Questioning, 94
Questionnaires, 74, 94–96

R

Range of motion, 120–121
Reflex-spasm model, 126
Rehabilitation, 35
  work related, 102–109
Relaxation training, 125–128
Reliability, 81
Rheumatic pain, 19
Risk factors, 15
  back pain, 15, 22–23, 37
Role
  checklist, 85
  loss of, 148

S

Scandinavia, 18–19
Self-care difficulties, 97–98
Self-efficacy beliefs, 64
Self-Efficacy Gauge, 64, 87
Self-efficacy measurement, 87
Self-help groups, 132–133
Sexual difficulties, 98–99
Skills
  coping, 130–132
  of occupational therapists, 156–162
Somatic pain, 147
Spinal disorders, 17
Spinothalamic tract, 9
Sports medicine, 35
Stress–causality model, 126–127
Stress management, 128–130
Substantia gelatinosa cells, 9
Survey of Pain Attitudes, 74
Survey of Pain Attitudes Revised (SOPAR), 86
Sympathetically maintained pain, 7

T

Therapeutic procedures, painful, 143
Transmission cells (T cells), 9
Traumatic paediatric pain, 142
Treatment see Management

U

United Kingdom
  occupational therapists in pain clinics, 49–50
  pain surveys, 17

United States of America
  back pain, 20, 48
  acute back pain occupational therapy program, 48
  chronic pain management program, 47–48
  pain surveys, 19–21
Uptime measurement, 96
Utility, 81

V

Validity, 81
Ventriculostomy, 33
Vicious cycles, 58
Visceral pain, 147
Visual Analogue Scale, 74, 148
Volition, 56
Volitional systems, 85–86, 160

W

Waddell Impairment Index, 79

West Haven Yale Multidimensional Pain Inventory (WHYMPI; MPI), 76–78, 145
WHO analgesic ladder, 32
Work, 99–109
  and chronic pain, 101
  and health, 101
  occupational history, 84–85
  occupational therapist's role, 102–107, 161
  rehabilitation, 102–109
  work-related back pain *see* Back pain: work-related
Work abilities assessment, 97
Work capacity evaluation (WCE), 104
Work disability model, 101
Work hardening, 105–106
Work tolerance screening (WTS), 104–105
Worksite (on-the-job) assessment, 107